A CAREGIVER'S GUIDE TO DEMENTIA

USING ACTIVITIES AND OTHER STRATEGIES TO PREVENT, REDUCE AND MANAGE BEHAVIORAL SYMPTOMS

LAURA N. GITLIN, Ph.D.

CATHERINE VERRIER PIERSOL, Ph.D., OTR/L

Camino Books, Inc.

Philadelphia

Manufactured in the United States of America

2 3 4 17 16 15

Library of Congress Cataloging in Publication Data

Gitlin, Laura N., 1952–
A caregiver's guide to dementia: using activities and other strategies to prevent, reduce and manage behavioral symptoms / Laura N. Gitlin, Ph.D., Catherine Verrier Piersol, Ph.D., OTR/L.
   pages cm
   ISBN 978-1-933822-90-7 (alk. paper)
  1. Dementia—Nursing. 2. Dementia—Patients—Care. 3. Caregivers. I. Piersol, Catherine Verrier, 1959– II. Title.

   RC521.G578 2014
   616.8'3—dc23   2014012067

   ISBN: 978-1-933822-90-7
   ISBN: 978-1-933822-91-4 (ebook)

Cover and interior design: Jerilyn Bockorick

For additional information, visit the Center for Innovative Care in Aging at:
www.nursing.jhu.edu/agingcenter and www.jefferson.edu/university/health_professions/elder_care

This book is available at a special discount on bulk purchases for promotion, business and educational use.

Publisher
Camino Books, Inc.
P.O. Box 59026
Philadelphia, PA 19102
www.caminobooks.com

Acknowledgments

The information provided in this guide was developed in part from research studies funded by the National Institutes of Health, Pennsylvania Department of Health, the Alzheimer's Association, and the Administration on Aging. We are grateful to the numerous people who contributed to the advancement of the strategies included in this guide including interventionists (occupational therapists) and family caregivers in our research studies. We would like to acknowledge in particular the contributions of Dr. Mary Corcoran and Tracey Vause Earland to initial drafts. The guide can be used by families and care providers by itself or as part of evidence-based caregiver education and skill-building programs.

The guide was developed by:

Laura N. Gitlin, Ph.D.

Professor, Department of Community Public Health
School of Nursing
Joint Appointments: Department of Psychiatry, Division of Geriatrics and Gerontology, School of Medicine
Director, Center for Innovative Care in Aging
Johns Hopkins University
http://nursing.jhu.edu/excellence/aging/center/index.html
agingcenter@jhu.edu

Catherine Verrier Piersol, Ph.D., OTR/L

Associate Professor, Department of Occupational Therapy
Clinical Director, Jefferson Elder Care
Jefferson School of Health Professions
Thomas Jefferson University
http://www.jefferson.edu/elder_care
eldercare@jefferson.edu

Recommended citation: Gitlin, L.N., and Piersol, C.V. *A Caregiver's Guide to Dementia: Using Activities and Other Strategies to Prevent, Reduce and Manage Behavioral Symptoms* (E-book, 2014).

The suggestions in this guide are intended for guidance and not to replace advice or directions given by a physician, therapist, or other health or human service professional. The author(s) disclaim liability for any injuries resulting in connection with the use of these tips, suggestions, or guidelines.

Contents

SECTION 8
Worksheets

Address Challenging Behaviors

Challenging Behaviors

One of the greatest challenges in caring for a person with dementia is preventing and managing behaviors. Behavioral symptoms are almost universal — they can occur at any stage of the disease and with any type of dementia. Most people with dementia will experience one or more behavioral symptoms as part of the course of the disease. Some behaviors can be dangerous or disturbing to the person with dementia and disruptive and frustrating to the people around them.

Using activities as part of daily care or on a regular basis can help prevent distressful behaviors from occurring or reduce the frequency of their occurrences. Other strategies may also be needed. It is unclear why behavioral symptoms that are atypical for the person occur. Some behaviors may be the result of brain damage from the disease. Whereas other behaviors may be prompted by multiple and co-occurring conditions that can be identified and then changed or modified. Conditions that can contribute to behaviors may be related to the person with dementia, such as an underlying medical condition, pain, poor sleep or feelings of insecurity; or conditions related to the caregiver such as when overly complex communications are used, or if the caregiver is stressed and overwhelmed; or conditions related to the physical environment, such as if there is too much or too little stimulation, too much clutter, poor lighting or poor ways of finding cues.

In the sections that follow, we consider common behaviors that families can find challenging, the possible factors, conditions or "triggers" that may be contributing to these behaviors, and specific ways or strategies to modify or eliminate these factors to help prevent or minimize the occurrences of behaviors. These strategies can be used in addition to or in combination with activities.

Common Triggers of Behavioral Symptoms

Triggers Related to the Person with Dementia

- Pain or discomfort due to an underlying medical condition
- Fatigue or lack of sleep
- Over-stimulation
- Under-stimulation or boredom
- Fright
- Confusion or disorientation
- Frustration
- Anxiety or worry
- Fearfulness
- Hunger
- Too hot or cold

Triggers Related to the Caregiver

- Stressed, overwhelmed, depressed
- Poor quality relationship with person with dementia
- Poor communication style
- Poor health

Triggers Related to the Environment

- Too little stimulation
- Too much stimulation
- Poor lighting
- Difficulty finding way
- Too much clutter
- Too hot or cold

Understanding, Identifying and Modifying Possible Triggers of Behaviors

Challenging behaviors may occur due to a medical issue. A medical condition should be considered especially if a behavior suddenly occurs or increases dramatically in frequency. It is important to ask the doctor of the person with dementia about whether the following factors may be contributing to behaviors you are observing:

What to Ask the Doctor:

- Could side effects of medications my family member is taking possibly contribute to the behavior?

- Could an interaction of several medications be causing the behavior?

- Does my family member have an infection such as a urinary tract infection or a sinus infection or other underlying medical condition (e.g., anemia) that may be contributing to the behavior?

- Could he/she be in pain or discomfort?

- Could he/she be suffering from dehydration or constipation?

- Could my family member have a vision or hearing problem that is making the behavior worse?

To help identify other potential triggers of a behavior, consider the setting in which it occurs. Ask yourself these questions:

- *Where* does the behavior occur?

- *When* does it occur?

- *How* frequently does it occur?

- *Who* is present when it occurs?

For example, does the behavior only happen when it is time to leave the home, time to eat or get dressed? By specifying these aspects of the behavior, you will be able to identify some of the triggers that may contribute to the behavior, and which can be modified. Consider keeping track of the behavior over a one- or two-week period using the *behavior tracking form*, which can be found in Section 8 of this guide.

Next, consider the result: What happens to you and the person with dementia as the behavior occurs or immediately after the behavior ends?

For example, do you become very upset? Do you express your anger or frustration? Does the person with dementia become even more agitated? It may be helpful to use the behavior tracking form to record what happens after the behavior occurs, as well as why you think the behavior occurred.

How might you address the behavior?

Based on the information you have gathered about what happens before, during, and after a behavior, the next step is to *brainstorm* possible strategies for preventing, reducing or addressing the behavior.

- "Brainstorming" is a method of solving specific problems by spontaneously thinking of new and creative ideas without immediately judging whether they will work or not. After you have brainstormed for 10 minutes or so, go back and critically look at your ideas and whether they are doable. You can brainstorm with a health-care professional or someone else you know who has experience with these problems. Here are some general guidelines for brainstorming:
  - Always work on one behavior at a time.
  - Consider what your personal goal is (e.g. prevent the behavior, minimize its occurrences, make it safer for the person if the behavior occurs.)
  - Consider which triggers can be changed.
  - Review the strategies provided in this guide.
  - Check off the specific strategies that will work best for you.

- Strategies are designed to help minimize the occurrence of the behavior or address the behavior when it occurs. The strategies may also help keep the person with dementia safe, comfortable and content; as well as preserve your own energy, time, patience and financial resources.

After brainstorming, try to implement one or more strategies:

- Try out the one(s) you have chosen.

- Try just one strategy at a time or try several, depending on the behavior.

- You may have to try a strategy for 1 to 2 weeks before you are able to notice a difference in the person with dementia's behavior.

- If you find that a strategy makes the behavior worse, discontinue it.

- You may benefit from working with a health professional to review your situation.

- Communication strategies are highly effective — so try these first.

Finally, evaluate whether the strategy is effective: Does it work?

- Record or monitor which strategies seem to reduce or help address the problem behavior.

- If the strategies do not work, then try others from your brainstorming list. You may also want to then talk to family members, health professionals and the doctor of the person you are caring for about the behavior to identify other strategies for addressing the behavior.

When to Seek Professional Help

In addition to using this guide and talking with the physician of the person with dementia, you may find it helpful to talk to other specialists. One such specialist is an occupational therapist with dementia care expertise who can help caregivers implement the strategies in this guide. Your doctor can provide you with a referral. What do occupational therapists do?

- Occupational Therapists (OTs) with dementia-related experience specialize in:
  - Evaluating the person with dementia's capabilities
  - Helping you establish a daily routine and use activities
  - Recommending changes to your home environment to make it safe for the person with dementia and easier for you to provide care
  - Identifying the specific strategies that may work best for your situation
  - Helping you reduce your stress and take care of yourself

- When to ask your doctor for a referral to occupational therapy:
  - You need help making your home safe for the person with dementia.
  - You need help implementing the strategies in this guide or modifying them to fit your situation.
  - The person with dementia continues to reject care or has difficulty with bathing, toileting, dressing, feeding or grooming.

- You are not sure if the person with dementia can be left alone.
- You need help planning a routine and/or getting time for yourself.
- You are unsure what the person with dementia is able to do.
- You need help identifying and using activities.
- You are not sure how to communicate effectively.
- You have back or neck strain due to lifting or transferring the person with dementia.

Use Activities
in Daily Care

Why Are Activities Important?

A person with dementia experiences many losses as the disease progresses including difficulties engaging in everyday activities such as work, driving, socializing, previous hobbies, or self-care in the same way as they did previously. As the disease progresses, it may become increasingly challenging for the person with dementia to think of an activity to participate in, know how to initiate the activity, problem-solve as to how to organize and set up the activity, follow a sequence of actions needed to engage in the activity, recognize errors and self-correct in carrying out the activity, or simply understand what to do. It is not uncommon for a person with dementia to experience boredom, frustration, agitation or depression as he/she loses cognitive abilities and as previously valued everyday activities become more difficult to engage in successfully.

Nevertheless, a person with dementia continues to need to be engaged and participate in daily life in meaningful ways throughout the course of the disease. Being involved in common activities can reinforce a person's sense of self-identity and provide meaning and purpose regardless of the stage of the disease. Helping a person with dementia maintain a sense of purpose and involvement in meaningful activities is an enduring need throughout the course of the disease.

It is important to identify ways of enabling a person with dementia to participate in activities that have meaning and interest to them. Helping a person with dementia to engage in an activity is a critical part of maintaining and/or enhancing their quality of life and should be part of a daily care approach. Activities may include everyday tasks such as dressing, bathing, preparing meals; or hobbies such as gardening, taking a walk, looking at meaningful photographs, exercising, sorting beads or coins, or other special interests such as listening to soothing music or watching a musical or other video of meaning.

Almost any activity can be set up in such a way as to enable a person with dementia at almost any level of cognitive functioning to effectively and meaningfully participate in it. Introducing activities that match to or fit with the person's interests and abilities can benefit both the person with dementia and their family caregiver.

What Are the Benefits of Activities?

Activities promote positive feelings and a sense of well-being in the person with dementia

Everyone needs to feel needed and useful. Engaging in daily tasks like folding laundry, or spending time in a fun, pleasant activity such as listening to music, sorting beads, or taking a walk, can provide a feeling of accomplishment and purpose. Being engaged is an important part of being a human being and having quality of life. Being engaged in activities provides a sense of self-worth and personal security and a positive sense of self.

Activities can improve mood and help prevent behaviors that may be disturbing to you and the person with dementia

When a person with dementia is unable to engage in an activity, he or she may become bored, frustrated, irritable or upset. Knowing what and how to introduce appropriate engaging activities can prevent these feelings and behaviors from occurring. Having a regular, predictable routine that involves participation in daily activity may improve the person's mood.

Activities can make caregiving easier

Engaging the person with dementia in activities that she/he enjoys can free time for yourself. Also, engaging with the person with dementia in an activity that is also enjoyable for you can make you feel good, too.

How to Use Activities in Daily Care

A person with dementia may need help in different ways to effectively engage in an activity. Here are some of the key areas for which a person with dementia may need help:

- Identifying an activity

- Setting up the activity

- Initiating the activity

- Knowing what to do or the steps of the activity

- Planning for the activity

- Organizing the activity

- Safely participating in the activity

- Knowing when to do the activity

By identifying which areas the person with dementia needs help with, you can help that person effectively engage in the activity. For example, if a person has difficulty initiating the activity, then you can use a verbal "prompt" or "cue" to help the person get started (Mom, here is our favorite photo album; let's look at the photos now). Consider the following step-by-step approach.

Step 1. Identify an Activity

- A person with dementia may require help identifying an activity to do, setting it up, following steps of the activity or knowing what to do.

- To identify an activity, think about what the person with dementia used to enjoy doing prior to the dementia or what you think the person might still like to do now. For example, if the person with dementia was a homemaker, then helping you develop a shopping list, folding towels or rolling socks may be a meaningful activity to use on a regular basis. If the person with dementia used to work with his/her hands, then perhaps sorting beads or coins, or participating in a craft such as painting, whittling or sanding a simple piece of wood may be engaging.

- Any activity can be modified or simplified to enable a person with dementia to participate in it. So don't worry about identifying an activity that you think may be too complex. Focus on identifying an activity that the person expressed he/she wants to do or you think she/he might enjoy as it may tap into previous interests, work or activities they used to participate in.

- For persons at the early stage of the disease, engage the person in a conversation about things they may like to try or what they like that they are presently doing. List a few activities you think they may have enjoyed in the past to guide the conversation.

- For persons at the moderate to moderate severe stage of the disease, consider activities that:
  - are highly familiar
  - involve large body movement (gross motor) such as wiping a table or washing windows
  - use simple and familiar objects (For example, if the person with dementia used to work at a desk, provide a notebook, a telephone message pad or checkbook for him/her to use.)
  - are repetitive (e.g., using a vacuum, placing beads from one container to another)
  - require one step directions
  - represent past interests or roles
  - are not competitive such as games
  - the rules can be relaxed (in a competitive game) as the person with dementia may not be able to follow the rules or play the way they used to, yet they may still derive enjoyment from participation
  - give preference to leisure or work outlets that are cooperative versus competitive

- For persons at the severe to end stage of the disease but who are still responsive to their environment, consider activities that are more passive such as listening to soothing music, watching a video of repetitive objects, animals, babies, or of nature. Also, consider tossing a balloon or simple chair exercises.

Step 2. Set Up the Environment for the Activity

- Identify an area in which the activity will occur. In selecting an area, consider the following:
  - Is the lighting adequate to engage in the activity?
  - Is the space adequate for the activity?
  - Is the chair or seating arrangement appropriate for the person to engage in the activity?

- Adjust the height of tables or chairs to optimally position the person with dementia. The best seated position is with feet flat on the floor, back straight, and table at waist level. A chair with armrests is also recommended for extra support. If the person with dementia's feet do not reach the floor, try putting a large book, such as a phone book, a box, or a footstool under his/her feet to provide support.

- Assure appropriate lighting. Install adequate lighting at the table, countertop, or work areas. As a person gets older his/her eyesight can become more sensitive to glare. Reduce glare by:
  - using polarized sunglasses for outdoor activities;
  - eliminating highly polished surfaces, especially floors;
  - placing a non-skid rug over bare floors under windows;
  - using light letters on a dark background for signs.

- Remove objects that are not necessary for the activity in the area in which it will be conducted so as not to distract the person with dementia.

- Put out one interesting item/game/activity where the person with dementia will notice.

- When interest decreases, replace with another activity of the appropriate skill level.

- Make sure to place any objects within sight of the person with dementia, as a reminder that these objects are available for them to use.

- If the activity is to "putter" freely or roam, simplify and make safe one area in the home, such as the living room, garage, or yard for the person with dementia.

- Use a screen or curtain to hide distracting items from view.

- If it is necessary to monitor the person with dementia, set up the activity in an area that will make supervision easier for you. For example, use the kitchen table for the activity as you prepare a meal.

- Put materials for an activity in an organizing bin for easy access and use. This will help you to set up the activity quickly and easily, which may be especially important if you are using the activity to distract the person or reduce agitation just before you notice it occurring or as it begins. The organization will also help the person with dementia to feel more at ease with the activity.

- Use "hot" colors to increase visibility of objects. Hot colors include yellows, oranges and reds. Avoid "cool" colors, which include greens and blues, as these colors become more difficult to see as a person ages and experiences changes in vision.

- Use dark colors and increase the size of letters, forms, or pictures used to communicate information to the person with dementia. Due to changes in vision and cognition, these techniques will help increase the person with dementia's ability to see and understand the information you present to him/her.

Step 3. Introduce the Activity

- To introduce the activity, do not physically pull or push to get the person with dementia to do what you want him/her to do. Try this approach:

- Move up behind and to the side of the person with dementia, take his or her elbow, and gently walk with him/her.
- Calmly state where both of you are going.
- If the person with dementia resists, do not force him/her to comply.
- Relax the rules and standards of the activity in order to provide a feeling of success. For example, do not worry if the bed is made incorrectly. Provide praise for his/her efforts and ignore mistakes.

- Establish successful experiences. Allow the person with dementia to win a game. Praise how a task was completed or the outcome. Comment about how great it is to have him/her help or be with you. Praise desirable behavior and ignore undesirable behavior. If undesirable behavior becomes intolerable, use distractions.

- Reduce the complexity of the activity on "bad" days. For example, there might be days when the person with dementia does not feel well or seems more confused. To make the activity easier, try:
  - Reducing the number of objects or choices. For example, if the person enjoys working with beads and has been sorting different colors, on a "bad" day, have them only sort 2 colors (black and white beads), or just move all the beads from one container to another.
  - Giving more verbal assistance
  - Simplifying the rules

Step 4. Enhance Engagement

- People with dementia vary in the level and type of assistance they may need to enable them to effectively engage in an activity. Through observation of the person you are caring for you may be able to identify what specifically they are having difficulty with. The person with dementia may have difficulty with one or more of the following areas:
  - Initiation — the individual has difficulty starting an activity
  - Sequencing — the individual has difficulty coordinating and ordering the steps involved in an activity
  - Organization — the individual has difficulty obtaining or arranging materials needed for the activity
  - Planning — the individual has difficulty determining how to do the activity and planning for its occurrence
  - Execution — the individual has difficulty carrying out the activity overall and exercising good judgment and safety
- Using verbal and nonverbal (such as gestures) strategies can help a person initiate, sequence, organize, plan and execute or perform an activity. These strategies are referred to as "cues" which are external supports that provide assistance to enable the person to successfully engage in an activity. External cues may include visual,

auditory and tactile information that can trigger the person with dementia to participate in an activity.

- Consider using types of cues or prompts.

Types of Cues or Prompts to Consider

No Cues Required:

The person with dementia does not need any cues to initiate, sequence, organize, execute or perform the activity safely.

Indirect Verbal Guidance:

The person with dementia at an early stage may need some verbal guidance such as an open-ended question:

> *"What should you do next?"*

Gestural Cue:

The person with dementia at a moderate disease stage may benefit from a nonverbal prompt such as a physical gesture that guides the participant, or pointing to where the person needs to go.

Tactile Cue:

The person with dementia at a mild, moderate or severe disease stage may need a tactile cue such as touching on the arm or gently leading him/her physically by the arm to where the activity will take place.

Direct Verbal Cue:

The person with dementia at a moderate to severe disease stage may need a one-step verbal command to either initiate, sequence, or fully execute or perform the activity. For example, *"put the bead in the container"*; *"turn on the water"*; *"pick up your toothbrush."*

Other Cues:

Some environmental cues may be helpful such as labeling objects, using big lettering or pictures of objects such as a picture of socks on the sock drawer.

With disease progression, you will need to simplify the activity. Refer to the strategies throughout this guide and then use the worksheets in Section 8 to record ways to simplify the activity.

Activities to Consider

Sorting activities:

- Poker chips, coins, beads, playing cards, plastic utensils
- Sort objects by shape, color or size.

Outdoor activities:

- Raking, washing windows, simple gardening, stringing cheerios to hang outside for the birds, sweeping the sidewalk or deck, wiping off patio furniture

Interactive activities:

- Toss a ball or balloon, play horseshoes, play with a child, look at photographs together, play with a pet, sing old songs or hymns, have afternoon tea, dance, finish famous sayings or bible quotations, play tick tac toe.

Repetitive arm movement activities:

- Fold towels or clothes, vacuum rugs, wipe off the table, sand wood, rub in hand lotion, sweep the floor, roll yarn into a ball, wash windows or a car, rake leaves.

"Window watching" activities:

- Allow the person with dementia to watch the activities of the neighborhood through the window or from the porch, as long as the person you are caring for is not disturbed by his or her observations.

Walking activities:

- Walking with another person is an excellent pastime for the person with dementia as long as the route is safe.
- Choose a circular route for walking because it is sometimes difficult to have the person with dementia turn around and change directions. If you must change directions, stop the person with dementia. Distract him/her by stopping to admire something, then casually start up again in the direction you want to go.

Other activities:

- Look through supermarket circulars or magazines, listen to music, color pictures, put a puzzle together, decorate paper placemats, arrange fresh flowers, sew sewing cards, wash lettuce, peel potatoes or carrots.

Traveling or short excursions as an activity

- To travel, evaluate how well the person with dementia handles small outings and changes in the daily routine. Irritability, extreme irritability or anxiety (catastrophic reactions), loss of appetite and difficulty sleeping all indicate that the outing was too disruptive to the person with dementia. Even if the person with dementia tolerates travel well, he/she may be more confused and edgy than usual when traveling.

- Preserve the daily routine as much as possible.

- Plan times for rest (3 rests plus meals would be optimal).

- Consider taking a third person along to help. Traveling can be more work than simply staying at home.

- Bring an "Occupied" sign to place on public rest rooms if the person with dementia needs help to toilet.

- Carry a recent photo of the person with dementia in case he/she gets lost. Also, make note of the clothing worn daily by the person with dementia and make sure he/she is carrying some form of identification. Place a card in his/her pocket with your name, name of the hotel, name of an emergency number at home, and the name of the tour if applicable.

- Plan to provide extra help with dressing and bathing because the surroundings will be unfamiliar and confusing.

- Keep travel plans flexible and arrival and departure dates open to accommodate the possibility that things do not proceed as anticipated.

- Be realistic. Vacations will not generally relax the person with dementia nor will he/she necessarily return "better off."

- If flying, notify the airport that you are traveling with an impaired individual.

- Keep a change of clothing and some "baby wipes" handy.

- Bring an object that provides comfort and familiarity.

General Tips for Using Activities

There is no right or wrong way

- As long as the person with dementia is safe, there is no right or wrong way of doing an activity. For example, it does not matter if the person with dementia does not follow the rules of a card game or paints outside the lines. What does matter is if the person is engaged and finding pleasure in the activity. Remember to relax the rules when using activity.

Engagement is the goal

- The goal of an activity is to be engaged. Being engaged has important psychological and health benefits. The goal should not be to learn something new or to improve memory. For example, when looking at a magazine or photo album, the goal is to have the person with dementia derive pleasure and be engaged in looking at or describing the pictures. The goal is not to jog the person's memory about current or past events or facts.

Do not expect too much

- If washing dishes is a fun activity for the person – let the person just enjoy washing. The dishes may not get clean but that is okay.

Activities should be part of daily routines

- Activities should be integrated into a highly structured daily routine for a person with dementia, particularly at the moderate to moderate severe stage of the disease. A predictable, structured daily routine helps a person with dementia know what is expected and to feel more in control. When using activities, introduce those that are more active in the morning to early afternoon; choose activities that are more quiet and sedentary in the late afternoon or early evening so that the person will be able to better prepare for bedtime.

Choose activities that have interest

- An activity must have interest to a person for positive engagement to occur. If an activity does not appear to have interest to the person, then try another activity. You will be able to tell if the person with dementia is interested in an activity and engaged. Common signs that the activity is of interest include: facial signs such as a smile, verbal expressions of pleasure, sitting quietly and attending to the activity, less agitation and upset, appears relaxed. A person with dementia may engage in an activity for a few minutes, get up and walk away and then come back to the activity. That is okay. This behavior may be that person's way of engaging; they may need a break or walk around before starting the activity again.

Determine if the activity is of interest

- If you think that the person with dementia would like a particular activity but they don't seem to want to engage in it, consider trying the activity another day. Maybe they are tired or do not want to participate when you first introduce the activity. Try the activity up to 3 different days/times to see if it is of interest. If not, consider whether the activity is of interest but too complex and needs to be simplified; consider whether the activity does not have any interest at all and should not be used; consider whether you have set up the activity in a way that effectively engages the person (Is there sufficient light? Is the chair comfortable?); consider the time of day (Is the person too hungry to participate in the activity?).

Do not rush an activity

- When using an activity, do not rush the process. A person with dementia may need more time starting and being engaged in an activity. Do not make the person feel rushed.

Stay calm and relaxed

- Creating a calm and relaxing environment is important to help the person with dementia also be calm and relaxed. If you are nervous, stressed, and/or in a rush, the person with dementia may feel similarly and become upset and agitated. Practice deep breathing or other stress reduction techniques to help manage how you are doing – this will help establish a supportive environment for engaging in activities.

Watch for upset or agitation

- You will be able to tell if a person is becoming upset, frustrated or agitated with the activity. If this occurs, then stop the activity and do not use it. The activity may be too complex for the person or it may be a bad day for the person.

Use simple activities

- Remember that the goal is engagement. A simple activity is best (e.g., sorting two color beads; or placing coins in a container, or folding towels) and can be a source of enjoyment for a person with dementia.

Try to include the person with dementia in everyday activities

- Consider ways to include the person with dementia in daily activities. For example, at meal time, the person with dementia can wash the lettuce, put pre-cut tomatoes or other salad items in the bowl, or toss the salad. The person may also be able to place the plates on the table with verbal instruction.

Give praise

- Be sure to let the person with dementia know what a great job they are doing. Also, let them know how much they are helping you.

Communicate Effectively

Communication Is Key

Having dementia can cause difficulties in how the person with dementia talks to and understands you. Remember to continue to communicate with the person with dementia, even if you cannot see or understand his or her responses. The disease is responsible for these difficulties. The person with dementia is not able to change the way he/she communicates; however, changing the way you communicate to the person with dementia can minimize some difficulties including behavioral challenges such as agitation, upset or distress in the person with dementia.

Communicating effectively is critical for the successful use of activities as well as preventing challenging behaviors or reducing their negative impact. Consider using these communication strategies for any type of activity from bathing or using the toilet to taking a walk or looking at a photo album. Practicing these positive communication strategies can make a big difference for you and the person with dementia.

Communicate with Words

Allow the person with dementia sufficient time to understand what you are saying and respond to you.

The person with dementia needs extra time for his/her brain to understand what you are saying.

- Speak slowly.

- Count to 5 (silently) after each phrase or each question you ask the person with dementia. This will allow time for the person with dementia to respond.

Use 1- or 2-step simple verbal commands.

This reduces the complexity of what you are asking the person with dementia to do.

- Break each task into very simple steps. This will make the task less overwhelming and make it easier for the person with dementia to participate.

- Use a very specific verbal prompt that clearly instructs the person with dementia to do an activity.

  For example, if you need to help the person with dementia stand up from the bed to walk to the bathroom, you might use the following verbal prompts one at a time:

  1. *Roll toward me.*

  2. *Sit up.*

  3. *Hold here* (point to bedpost).

  4. *Stand up.*

Avoid using prompts that are not specific enough.

- For example, **do not say:** *"Go get dressed," "Go do something relaxing,"* or *"Get ready for bed."* These prompts do not tell the person with dementia exactly how to get dressed, how to engage in an activity or what is needed in order to get ready for bed.

- Instead be more direct, do say: *"Put on your shirt," "Let's sit here,"* or *"Put on your pajama top."*

Give simple choices and no more than 2 choices at a time.

Giving the person with dementia a choice may give him/her a sense of personal control:

- Provide "either/or" choices.

- **Do not say:** *"What do you want for breakfast?"*

- Do say: *"Do you want Cheerios* (point to cheerios) *or eggs* (point to eggs) *for breakfast?*

Use the following words frequently when interacting with the person with dementia.

- *"Take your time, you can do this"* — Encourage the person with dementia with positive statements.

- *"Good job"* — Validate the person with dementia's actions.

- *"Everything is OK"* or *"it's OK, I locked all the doors and windows"* — Use calming words.

These words help to support and reassure the person with dementia.

Avoid using negative words and negative approaches.

Such words can make the person with dementia upset or agitated.

Avoid the Following Approaches	Avoid Saying
• Arguing	• *"You make me so angry."*
• Trying logic	• *"Why are you so stubborn?"*
• Scolding, yelling or talking loudly	• *"Why are you being mean today?"*
• Showing anger	• *"You're not being nice."*
• Making fun	

Identify yourself and others

If you are not sure the person with dementia will remember your name or the names of other family member and friends:

- This helps the person with dementia feel more at ease.

- Tell the person with dementia who you are when you walk up to him/her.

- Introduce a guest or other family member.

- Address the person with dementia by name. This helps focus his/her attention on you.

Go along with the person with dementia's belief of what is true and avoid arguing or trying to convince.

- It will frustrate you and the person with dementia and make the situation worse. You cannot win an argument. You can use his/her view to your advantage and he/she will feel safer and more assured.

- For example, do not tell the person with dementia that a loved one has been dead for years. The person with dementia will become more upset. Say something that will address his/her need and keep her calm. Say *"Your mother can't come today,"* or *"Your mother is safe."*

- Or if a person with dementia insists that her husband, who died 10 years ago, is coming to see her today. Tell her that if he is coming, she needs to get ready by getting out of bed and getting dressed.

Help the person with dementia find words to express him/herself.

- When the person with dementia is having difficulty expressing a thought, you may be able to guess what he or she is trying to say. Ask the person with dementia if you are guessing correctly. For example, say *"Are you worried about catching the bus to the center?"* or *"Are you saying you..."*

Eliminate noise and distractions while you are communicating.

- The person with dementia may not be able to "tune out" other sounds in the background while you are speaking to him or her. This may make it difficult for the person with dementia to concentrate on and understand what you are saying. For example, turn off the television or radio and never leave both on at the same time.

Communicate without Words

Use these strategies in combination with verbal strategies:

- Use a light touch to reassure, calm or redirect the person with dementia. For example, take the person with dementia's arm and direct him/her to where you want to go.

- Be aware of your facial expressions. Use smiles to provide encouragement and avoid frowning or showing anger or upset in your face.

- Use other signals other than words to help direct the person with dementia. Signals could include pointing, touching, or handing the person with dementia things.

- Make eye contact but do not stare. The person with dementia one may interpret prolonged eye contact as threatening or disturbing.

- Move slowly and calmly. Slow and steady movements allow your loved one more time to process and understand your actions. Moving quickly may contribute to agitation and/or confusion.

- Try to identify ways in which the person with dementia is using non-verbal messages to communicate with you.

  For example:

  - Repeated visits to the kitchen may be a sign that the person with dementia is hungry.

  - A sad face may indicate that the person with dementia is unhappy or uncomfortable about his/her surroundings or clothing.

  - Laughter and smiling can suggest that the person with dementia is happy and enjoying his/her current activity.

  - Grabbing at clothes or taking them off may mean the person with dementia is feeling too hot.

Use simple visual reminders.

- Tape an arrow on the wall to direct the person with dementia to the bathroom.

- Place a photo of a toilet on the bathroom door used by the person with dementia.

- Put a picture of what is in cabinets or drawers. An example for a bedroom dresser would be putting a picture of the type of clothing that is in each drawer for easier recognition.

Use simple written instructions.

- If the person with dementia can follow simple written instructions, use notes as a reminder for what the person with dementia should do. For example, place a sign above the sink or bathroom mirror saying:

  - Brush teeth

  - Wash your face

  - Comb hair

Express affection.

- Smile. Take the person with dementia's hand. Put your arm around his or her waist or in some other physical way express affection. Holding hands, hugging, and just sitting together are important ways to communicate.

Use Cues or Prompts to Enhance Participation in Activities

- If the person with dementia no longer understands verbal directions, use cueing. A cue is a signal, such as a word or action, used to prompt performance. A cue can be a verbal command, a visual prompt, or a tactile/physical prompt such as gently guiding the body through the movement.

- The person with dementia may need one or more of these "cues" from you to assist them in performing a given task. Whatever cue you use, be sure to allow the person with dementia sufficient time to understand and process your instruction. The person with dementia needs extra time for his/her brain to understand what you are communicating.

- A person may respond differently to various cues. Here are cueing strategies that may be helpful for initiating an action:
  - Begin with VERBAL cues.
  - If this is not successful, proceed to VISUAL cues.
  - If the person with dementia no longer responds to verbal and/or visual cueing alone, TACTILE cueing may be necessary to reduce frustration.

Try These Cueing Strategies for Any Activity:

Verbal Cueing

- Use 1 or 2 simple verbal commands. Use very specific verbal prompting that clearly instructs the person with dementia to do an activity. For example, if you need to help the person with dementia stand up from the bed to walk to the bathroom, you might use the following verbal cues one at a time:
  - Roll toward me.
  - Sit up.
  - Hold the bedpost.
  - Stand up.
  - Validate the person with dementia's action (e.g., *"good job"*).
  - Speak slowly.

Visual Cueing

- Limit the amount of words you use to direct the person with dementia. At some point in the illness, language is confusing for the individual with dementia and they have difficulty processing the words.

- Use signals other than words to help direct the person with dementia. Signals include pointing, touching or handing the person with dementia things. For example, point to the spoon right before the person with dementia reaches for the wrong utensil. Or, tap on the drinking glass to get the person with dementia's attention to drink.

- Demonstration may also serve as a visual cue for the person with dementia. Position yourself within his/her visual field so that they can observe you drinking from the glass. The person with dementia may imitate your actions.

Tactile Cueing

- If verbal and visual cueing is unsuccessful, try tactile cueing. Some people with dementia work best when they are provided with gentle physical assistance to complete an action. Hand-over-hand assistance may provide just enough information to the nervous system so that the person with dementia can successfully complete the task.

- Using a light touch, place your hand over the person with dementia's hand (holding the spoon) and initiate the motion of self-feeding. Hand-over-hand cueing serves as a reminder/prompt for the person with dementia.

- Move slowly and calmly, do not rush. Reassure the person with dementia that they are doing a good job.

Additional Points to Keep in Mind When Using Cues

- Allow the person with dementia sufficient time to respond to you.

- Avoid using negative words and negative approaches (do not scold or argue, or raise your voice).

- Eliminate noise and distraction while you are communicating (turn off the radio or TV).

- Be aware of your facial expressions, make eye contact but do not stare.

- Express affection — smile, hold hands, give a hug.

Make the Home Safe

Home Safety

People with dementia spend most of their time in their home or that of a family member with nothing to do. Engaging the person in activity and keeping the home safe becomes increasingly important with the progression of the disease. As the person with dementia's behavior and abilities change over time, it is important to periodically conduct a room-by-room inspection of your home to assure that it is safe for the person with dementia. It is difficult to know what a person with dementia might do. Just because something has not yet occurred does not mean it may not in the near future. Checking the safety of your home will help you take control of some of the potential problems that may create hazardous situations.

A safe home can be a less stressful home for the person with dementia, you and other family members.

The strategies we provide here are from our research, practice with families and a booklet from the Alzheimer's Disease Education Referral Center (ADEAR), which you may find helpful and which you can access freely on the Internet (Home Safety for People with Alzheimer's Disease):

http://www.nia.nih.gov/alzheimers/publication/home-safety-people-alzheimers-disease/introduction

Keep in mind these general points as you think about home safety and make changes to your home:

- It may not be necessary to make all of the changes suggested in the following pages. There can be a wide range of safety concerns that may arise, but some modifications may never be needed. Each home is unique and presents its own safety challenges. Consider the recommendations in the following pages as a guide.

- Your home is a personal and important environment to you, your family members and the person with dementia. As you consider changing your home, think about how the change may impact you and others and whether the change will be positive for everyone or be inconvenient or undesirable. It may be necessary to strike a balance. There are ways to make the home safe that will not disrupt others in the home. For example, removing objects or "decluttering" can be helpful to a person with dementia and less confusing to them. However, you may want to create a space just for you if you can that is off-limits to anyone else and arranged exactly as you like. Everyone needs private, quiet time, and you may find this helpful to you.

- Changing the environment can effectively address many behaviors. By making the home safe, you can decrease stressors in the environment that may be contributing to behavioral changes.

- By making the home safe and minimizing danger, you can help the person with dementia better move around the home safely and independently.

Is It Safe to Leave the Person with Dementia Alone?

Whether to leave a person with dementia alone needs careful evaluation, and you should discuss this with a health provider caring for that person. As abilities decline over time, constant reevaluation of home safety and being able to stay alone is necessary. The following questions (excerpted from the Alzheimer's Disease Education and Referral Center) may help you to evaluate whether it is safe to leave the person in a room alone or at home alone.

Does the person with dementia:

- become confused, upset or unpredictable under stress?
- recognize a dangerous situation, for example, fire?
- know how to use the telephone in an emergency?
- know how to get help?
- wander and become disoriented?
- show signs of agitation, depression or withdrawal when left alone for any period of time?
- attempt to cook, use sharp objects (for example for woodworking or other activities) that now require supervision?

Also, seek input and advice from a health care professional to assist you in these considerations. As dementia progresses, review these questions and continually evaluate the safety of the person you are caring for. Any change in behavior, function, or cognitive ability should trigger a reevaluation of home safety.

Use the following to help you identify potential hazards and to keep a record of changes you may need to make throughout your home.

General Safety Considerations

- Display emergency numbers and your home address near all telephones.
- Use an answering machine when you cannot answer phone calls, and set it to turn on after the fewest number of rings possible. A person with dementia often may be unable to take messages or could become a victim of telephone exploitation. Turn ringers on low to avoid distraction and confusion. Put all portable and cell phones and equipment in a safe place so they will not be easily lost.
- Install smoke alarms and carbon monoxide detectors in or near the kitchen and all sleeping areas. Check their functioning and batteries frequently.
- Avoid using flammable and volatile compounds near gas appliances. Do not store these materials in an area where a gas pilot light is used.

SECTION 4

- Install secure locks on all outside doors and windows.

- Hide a spare house key outside in case the person with dementia locks you out of the house.

- Avoid the use of extension cords if possible by placing lamps and appliances close to electrical outlets. Tack extension cords to the baseboards of a room to avoid tripping.

- Cover unused electrical outlets with childproof plugs.

- Place red tape around floor vents, radiators, and other heating devices to deter the person with dementia from standing on or touching them when hot.

- Check all rooms for adequate lighting.

- Place light switches at the top and the bottom of stairs.

- Stairways should have at least one handrail that extends beyond the first and last steps. If possible, stairways should be carpeted or have safety grip strips.

- Keep all medications (prescription and over-the-counter) locked. Each bottle of prescription medicine should be clearly labeled with the person's name, name of the drug, drug strength, dosage frequency and expiration date. Child-resistant caps are available if needed.

- Keep all alcohol in a locked cabinet or out of reach of the person with dementia. Drinking alcohol can increase confusion.

- If smoking is permitted, monitor the person with dementia while he or she is smoking. Remove matches, lighters, ashtrays, cigarettes, and other means of smoking from view. This reduces fire hazards, and with these reminders out of sight, the person may forget the desire to smoke. Do not let the person with dementia smoke alone.

- Avoid clutter, which can create confusion and danger. Throw out or recycle newspapers and magazines regularly. Keep all areas where people walk free of furniture.

- Keep plastic bags out of reach. A person with dementia may choke or suffocate.

- Remove all guns and other weapons from the home or lock them up. Install safety locks on guns or remove ammunition and firing pins.

- Lock all power tools and machinery in the garage, workroom or basement.

- Remove all poisonous plants from the home. Check with local nurseries or contact the poison control center for a list of poisonous plants.

- Make sure all computer equipment and accessories, including electrical cords, are kept out of the way. If valuable documents or materials are stored on a home computer, protect the files with passwords and back up the files.

- Passwords protect access to the Internet, and restrict the amount of online time without supervision. Consider monitoring computer use by the person with dementia, and install software that screens for objectionable or offensive material on the Internet.

- Keep fish tanks out of reach. The combination of glass, water, electrical pumps and potentially poisonous aquatic life could be harmful to a curious person with dementia.

Outside the Home

- Keep steps sturdy and textured to prevent falls in wet or icy weather.

- Mark the edges of steps with bright or reflective tape.

- Consider installing a ramp with handrails as an alternative to the steps.

- Eliminate uneven surfaces or walkways, hoses, and other objects that may cause a person to trip.

- Restrict access to a swimming pool by fencing it with a locked gate, covering it, and closely supervising it when in use.

- In the patio area, remove the fuel source and fire starters from any grills when not in use, and supervise use when the person with dementia is present.

- Place a small bench or table by the entry door to hold parcels while unlocking the door.

- Make sure outside lighting is adequate. Light sensors that turn on lights automatically as you approach the house may be useful. They also may be used in other parts of the home.

- Prune bushes and foliage well away from walkways and doorways.

- Consider a "NO SOLICITING" sign for the front gate or door.

Inside the Home

Entryway

- Remove scatter rugs and throw rugs.

- Use textured strips or nonskid wax on hardwood and tile floors to prevent slipping.

Kitchen

- Install childproof door latches on storage cabinets and drawers designated for breakable or dangerous items. Lock away all household cleaning products, matches, knives, scissors, blades, small appliances, and anything valuable.

- If prescription or nonprescription drugs are kept in the kitchen, store them in a locked cabinet.

- Remove scatter rugs and foam pads from the floor.

- Install safety knobs and an automatic shut-off switch on the stove.

- Do not use or store flammable liquids in the kitchen. Lock them in the garage or in an outside storage unit.

- Keep a night-light in the kitchen.

- Remove or secure the family "junk drawer." A person with dementia may eat small items such as matches, hardware, erasers and plastics.

- Remove artificial fruits and vegetables or food-shaped kitchen magnets, which might appear to be edible.

- Insert a drain trap in the kitchen sink to catch anything that may otherwise become lost or clog the plumbing.

- Consider disconnecting the garbage disposal. People with dementia may place objects or their own hands in the disposal.

Bedroom

- Anticipate the reasons a person with dementia might get out of bed, such as hunger, thirst, going to the bathroom, restlessness, and pain. Try to meet these needs by offering food and fluids and scheduling ample toileting.

- Use a night-light.

- Use a monitoring device (like those used for infants) to alert you to any sounds indicating a fall or other need for help. This also is an effective device for bathrooms.

- Remove scatter rugs and throw rugs.

- Remove portable space heaters. If you use portable fans, be sure that objects cannot be placed in the blades.

- Be cautious when using electric mattress pads, electric blankets, electric sheets, and heating pads, all of which can cause burns and fires. Keep controls out of reach.

- If the person with dementia is at risk of falling out of bed, place mats next to the bed, as long as they do not create a greater risk of accident.

- Use transfer or mobility aids when moving the person with dementia from one surface to another, as from the bed to the commode.

- If you are considering using a hospital-type bed with rails and/or wheels, read the Food and Drug Administration's up-to-date safety information at http://www.fda.gov/MedicalDevices/ProductsandMedicalProcedures/GeneralHospitalDevicesandSupplies/HospitalBeds/default.htm.

Bathroom

- Do not leave a severely impaired person with dementia alone in the bathroom.

- Remove the lock from the bathroom door to prevent the person with dementia from getting locked inside.

- Place nonskid adhesive strips, decals, or mats in the tub and shower. If the bathroom is uncarpeted, consider placing these strips next to the tub, toilet and sink.

- Use washable wall-to-wall bathroom carpeting to prevent slipping on wet tile floors.

- Use a raised toilet seat with handrails, or install grab bars beside the toilet.

- Install grab bars in the tub/shower. A grab bar in contrasting color to the wall is easier to see.

- Use a foam rubber faucet cover (often used for small children) in the tub to prevent serious injury should the person with dementia fall.

- Use a plastic shower chair or bath bench and a hand-held shower head to make bathing easier.

- In the shower, tub and sink, use a single faucet that mixes hot and cold water to avoid burns.

- Set the water heater at 120°F to avoid scalding tap water.

- Insert drain traps in sinks to catch small items that may be lost or flushed down the drain.

- Store medications (prescription and nonprescription) in a locked cabinet. Check medication dates and throw away outdated medications.

- Remove cleaning products from under the sink, or lock them away.

- Use a night-light.

- Remove small electrical appliances from the bathroom. Cover electrical outlets.

- If a man with dementia uses an electric razor, have him use a mirror outside the bathroom to avoid water contact.

Living Room

- Clear electrical cords from all areas where people walk.

- Remove scatter rugs or throw rugs. Repair or replace torn carpet.

- Place decals at eye level on sliding glass doors, picture windows or furniture with large glass panels to identify the glass pane.

- Do not leave the person with dementia alone with an open fire in the fireplace. Consider alternative heating sources.

- Keep matches and cigarette lighters out of reach.

- Keep the remote controls for the television, DVD player and stereo system out of sight.

Laundry Room

- Keep the door to the laundry room locked if possible.

- Lock all laundry products in a cabinet.

- Remove large knobs from the washer and dryer if the person with dementia tampers with machinery.

- Close and latch the doors and lids to the washer and dryer to prevent objects from being placed in the machines.

Garage/Shed/Basement

- Lock access to all garages, sheds and basements if possible.

- Inside a garage or shed, keep all potentially dangerous items, such as tools, tackle, machines and sporting equipment, either locked away in cabinets or in appropriate boxes/cases.

- Secure and lock all motor vehicles and keep them out of sight if possible. Consider covering vehicles, including bicycles, that are not frequently used. This may reduce the possibility that the person with dementia will think about leaving.

- Keep all toxic materials, such as paint, fertilizers, gasoline or cleaning supplies, out of view. Either put them in a high, dry place, or lock them in a cabinet.

- If the person with dementia uses the garage, shed or basement (preferably with supervision), make sure the area is well lit and that stairs have a handrail and are safe to walk up and down. Keep walkways clear of debris and clutter, and place overhanging items out of reach.

Support Health of the Person with Dementia

Be a Medical Advocate

People with dementia may have health risks and physical difficulties, but they may no longer be able to reliably report how they are feeling, describe their symptoms, or communicate effectively with the doctor. As the person providing care, you may have to assume the role of medical advocate for the person you are caring for. Monitoring health can also help to keep the person with dementia engaged in activities. It is important to organize and record important medical information about the person you care for.

When talking to the doctor of the person you care for, here are 5 critical issues you should be aware of:

1. Medication-related problems (like drug interactions or the use of drugs that interfere with memory or increase confusion)

- Be sure to ask the doctor to review all medications that are taken by the person you care for, and whether the dose or different combination of medications may be contributing to a worsening of behavior or other condition.

2. Dehydration (especially in hot weather)

- Ask the doctor how to prevent dehydration in the person you care for.

- Ask the doctor if the person you care for could be dehydrated, and whether this may be contributing to a worsening of behavior or other condition.

3. Constipation

- Ask the doctor how to prevent constipation in the person you care for.

- Ask the doctor if the person you care for could be constipated, and whether this may be contributing to a worsening of behavior or other condition.

4. Incontinence

- Ask your doctor to see if any of the medicines being taken by the person you care for could be causing incontinence. The physician may be able to prescribe medications that can help control it.

5. Pain (from undetected infections or injuries)

- Ask the doctor of the person you care for if he or she could be in pain or physical discomfort, which may be contributing to a worsening of behavior or other condition.

About Medications

Although medicine is intended to help, it can hurt if the person with dementia takes too much or mixes medicines that do not go together. Many people are harmed each year by taking the wrong medicine or the wrong combination of medicines.

You can obtain the best results for the person with dementia you are caring for by being a well-informed partner with the doctor and pharmacist. Follow these suggestions when talking with the doctor of the person you are caring for:

- Tell the doctor about ALL the medicines the person with dementia is taking. This includes over-the-counter medicines (like aspirin, laxatives and antihistamines), vitamins, herbal remedies (like St. John's wort and gingko biloba) and dietary supplements. Always take an updated, current list of medicines and their dosing with you to doctor appointments.

- Tell the doctor if the person with dementia has medicine allergies or has a history of problems taking particular medicines.

- Tell the doctor about other doctors or health care professionals who have prescribed medicine for the person with dementia or who have suggested a vitamin or herbal supplement.

- Tell the doctor about other illnesses or medical conditions the person with dementia may have, like diabetes or high blood pressure.

- If cost is a concern, there may be another medicine that costs less and will work the same.

- Get the facts about the medications that is being taken by the person with dementia. Make sure you know the following about each medicine:
  - What is the brand name and generic name of the medicine?
  - Can he/she take a generic version of this medicine?
  - What is he/she taking this medicine for?
  - Does this new prescription mean he/she should stop taking any other medicines being taken now?

- Write your questions down ahead of time. Take the list with you to appointments.

- Take notes when you get information from healthcare providers.

Other Tips

- Use the same pharmacy to buy all of your medicines so your prescription records will all be in one place.

- Read and save the patient information that comes with your medicine, often stapled to the bag from the pharmacy.

- Keep a list of all medicines, vitamins and dietary supplements that the person with dementia is taking. Add new medicines to the list.

Dehydration

- As the person caring for a person with dementia, you may need to be extra careful to make sure the person they are caring for does not become overheated or dehydrated when temperatures rise. In general, the elderly are more susceptible to health problems caused by heat, and people with dementia may be even more susceptible because it can be difficult for them to get the liquids that they need to keep hydrated. Dehydration is a major cause of hospitalization for the elderly.

- Prevention is key since mild dehydration has no symptoms. Dehydration is a risk with older adults for a number of reasons, including the following:
  - A reduced sense of thirst (if you are not thirsty, you drink less).
  - Diarrhea and/or vomiting.
  - Use of "water pills" (diuretics) with no replacement of water loss.
  - Disregard for a dry mouth (a common side effect of many drugs).
  - Fluid restrictions or simple forgetfulness.
  - If they leak urine or have to go to the bathroom frequently, they may think that drinking less will mean fewer trips to the bathroom or less leaking.
  - Insufficient fluids can increase the risks of constipation, loss of muscle strength, confusion and disorientation, urinary tract infections, pneumonia and pressure sores or ulcers.

- Judging a person's fluid needs is important. Set a goal of drinking 6 to 8 glasses a day. Fluid can include ice cream, Jell-O, and soup broth.

Factors That Increase Risk of Dehydration

- The thirst response, a normal protective mechanism to prevent dehydration, is lost with aging, especially in persons with dementia. Many medications also decrease thirst. The need for fluids will increase with fever or infection, low humidity, hot temperatures, losses due to diarrhea or vomiting. Patients with pulmonary diseases such as chronic obstructive pulmonary disease (COPD), emphysema or chronic bronchitis will lose additional fluids because of their increased breathing rate. Diabetes mellitus, if not adequately controlled, will result in additional loss of fluids.

- Mild dehydration has no symptoms, and even the symptoms of a more severe situation are not enough to offer a clear idea of the problem.

Signs of Possible Dehydration

- dry mouth (also a side effect of many drugs)

- decreased tears, dry or sunken eyes

- decreased urination and a darker-appearing, stronger-smelling urine, or constipation

- swollen or cracked tongue

- weight loss or muscle weakness

- skin that has lost its elasticity and feels "doughy"

- lightheadedness upon standing, due to low blood pressure

- decreased ability to perform normal activities

- falls or confusion

How Can You Increase Fluid Intake?

- Offer a variety of choices and avoid the use of beverages containing caffeine (tea, coffee, cola) or alcohol, which causes fluid losses. Remind the person you are caring for to drink something many times during the day. Don't offer too many confusing choices at any one time. To prevent boredom, offer a variety of drinks during the day.

- Give the person a drink first thing in the morning. Remember that they have been without fluids for as long as 12 hours and are probably very thirsty. Give more fluids with medication—about 6 ounces.

- Make fluids fun! Try offering mock cocktails and root beer floats.

Adapted from *Managing Nutrition in Dementia Care: A Supportive Approach for Caregivers,* Western New York Chapter of the Alzheimer's Association.

Constipation and Bowel Management

- The term constipation refers to difficulty with, and infrequent use of the bowels. What is normal varies from person to person, but as a rule, if a person goes three days without a bowel movement, or has difficulty or pain associated with hard bowel movement, they may well be constipated. Constipation is not a disease but a symptom of some underlying condition. A person who does not have dementia would soon recognize if he or she were constipated, and would eat some extra fruit or drink more fluids to alleviate the condition.

- The person with dementia may not recognize the problem but just feel discomfort when straining while on the toilet, and then stop. It is possible that some bowel fluid may be passed at this stage and that the caregiver thinks the person has diarrhea. The person may go to the toilet frequently, but not actually do anything. Constipation may cause hemorrhoids or small tears that become painful and further stop the person from using their bowels. They may become very embarrassed, especially if they accidentally soil their clothes or sheets. They may even try to conceal the evidence by wrapping it up in paper and hiding it in a drawer. This is not a purposeful action and needs to be handled in a tactful manner without punishing the person.

Some Likely Causes of Constipation

- **Diets low in fiber** may be related to sore gums, loss of teeth, poorly fitting dentures or life-long patterns of eating. Offer a well-balanced diet including whole-grain breads, fruit and vegetables if possible. Cut them up and offer as finger foods throughout the day. Visit a dentist regularly.

- **Lack of fluids other than coffee and tea.**
  Include some fruit juice or water and aim for 6 glasses per day.

- **Not enough exercise.**
  Try to go for a walk each day. Even just a walk through the garden for a few minutes is good. Do not overdo the walk; make it pleasurable so that the person wants to go.

- **Not recognizing or able to find the toilet.**
  Leave a door open, or label the door with the word "TOILET" in large print and/or a picture of a toilet.

- **Certain medications.**
  Check with a doctor if you think medication may be a cause.

- **Pain,** such as back pain, may make it impossible for the person to sit on the toilet. Ensuring that the toilet is the correct height, or that a footstool is being used, may prevent or ease pain.

- **New environment (e.g., holidays, hospital stay, friends visiting).**
  Ensure that the person knows where the toilet is in a new environment and that their usual habits are adhered to (e.g., going to the toilet at a regular time each day).

- **Fear,** particularly if it is dark. Leave a night-light on in the toilet or passageways.

- **Illness,** particularly if associated with fever and/or prolonged bed rest.

- **Poor bowel habits.**
  If possible, try to establish a routine and allow time for the person to sit. It may be beneficial to give a hot drink a short while prior to going.

- **Laxatives can be habit-forming** and should only be taken under a doctor's supervision.

- **Communication difficulties** may result in the person not being able to tell what the problem is even if they know. Memory difficulties may lead to the person saying they have used their bowel when in fact they have not

- **It may take time to improve the situation.**
  Keeping a good record of the bowel movements of the person you are caring for will assist you in treating the condition.

Adapted from: www.dementiacareaustralia.com/highlights.html

Managing Incontinence

- Incontinence is the loss of bladder or bowel control. Aging in itself causes changes in the urinary tract, which can lead to incontinence. Many different conditions and disorders can also cause incontinence, including dementia and neurological diseases.

- While there is no "cure" for incontinence, several habits can minimize symptoms and therefore lead to better bladder control. As with any health-related problem, it is always best to consult your doctor for help with treatment.

Dietary Habits

- A common mistake is reducing the amount of liquid a person consumes. While this does lead to less urine, the smaller amount of urine will be irritating to the bladder, increasing the risk of infection and further incontinence. **Instead, try to avoid these foods and drinks: beverages containing alcohol and caffeine, soft drinks, tomatoes and tomato-based products, spicy foods, sugar, honey and chocolate.** It is best for the person you are caring for to drink water.

Behavioral Habits

Use time toileting

- Set up a schedule for the person you are caring for to use the bathroom. His or her bladder is constantly being emptied, and there will be less chance of an accident. Toileting every 2 to 4 hours is recommended.

Clothing

- The person you are caring for should wear clothing that is easy to remove when it is time to use the toilet. Women should avoid nylon underpants and pantyhose. Cotton underpants are preferable, as they are the least irritating.

Smoking

- Smoking can increase intra-abdominal pressure (and therefore increased pressure on the bladder). It also increases bladder cancer risk.

Location, location, location

- Make sure that toilet facilities are convenient for your care recipient. Keep a bedside commode, bedpan or urinal nearby so that there is less distance to travel to a nearby toilet. Have the person you are caring for use the bathroom before leaving home for an appointment. If you are in a strange place, find the bathroom right away; don't wait until the person has to go and then try to find the bathroom.

Medical Considerations

Medication

- Ask the doctor if any of the medicines that the person you are caring for is taking could be causing incontinence. Even something as simple as an over-the-counter cold remedy can cause incontinence, so work with your doctor to see if you can switch medicines. Also, he or she can prescribe medications that can help control incontinence.

Surgery

- All appropriate nonsurgical treatments should be tried before considering surgery. There are different kinds of procedures that deal with different types of incontinence, so make sure to thoroughly discuss all of your options with your physician.

Devices

- Devices like catheters, pelvic support devices, urethral inserts or patches, external collection systems, penile compression devices and absorbent products are also available to help manage incontinence.

Take Care
of Yourself

Caring for a person with dementia can be an exhausting job physically and emotionally. Many families providing care put aside their own needs, leaving themselves at high risk for stress, poor health and other potential consequences. However, your needs are very important, and you have a duty to take care of yourself. Helping yourself stay as emotionally and physically healthy as you can while caring for a person with dementia is the best thing that you can do for you and the person you care for.

One important way of taking care of yourself is to manage the stressors of providing 24/7 care. Caregiving is hard work, and behaviors associated with dementia can be very upsetting and challenging to manage. The person you care for may not understand how you are feeling, but may nevertheless sense that you are upset or feel stressed. This, in turn, can make the person with dementia unhappy, agitated or worried. By managing your stress, you are also helping the person with dementia. One way of managing stress is to practice and use simple stress reduction techniques. Stress reduction techniques can help you manage the consequences of a behavior, or the frustration and upset you may feel providing care or responding to a challenging behavior. Another way to take care of yourself is to know how to protect yourself if the person you care for becomes physically combative (see the section on Aggressive or Combative Behaviors). Here we discuss stress and present a simple stress reduction technique for you to consider using on a regular basis.

What Is Stress?

Stress can be either short-term (acute) or long-term (chronic). Short-term or *acute stress* is a reaction to an immediate threat, commonly known as the "fight or flight" response. The threat can be any situation that is experienced as a danger. Examples can be as different as hearing a loud noise or having an infection. The physical response to stressors includes the release of stress hormones that produce an increased heart rate, blood pressure and muscle tension. Once the acute stress has passed, the response to the threat fades away and the levels of stress hormones return to normal. This is called the *relaxation response.*

Long-term or *chronic stress* is a reaction to ongoing stressful situations such as caregiving for someone for a long period of time. In a long-term stressful situation, the body stays tense and does not experience the relaxation response. Thus, blood pressure may stay elevated and the muscles may stay tense for a long period of time.

What are the consequences of chronic stress?

Psychological

- Stress can diminish your quality of life by reducing feelings of pleasure and accomplishment. It can lead to depression or anxiety, as well as feelings of anger and irritability.

Physical

- Stress over a long period of time can also affect you physically. Stress increases the risk of infections, heart disease and immune disorders. It can also lead to gastrointestinal and eating problems, sexual dysfunction, sleep disturbances and headaches.

Cognitive

- Stress can have an effect on memory, concentration and learning.

Social

- Long-term stress due to caregiving may also have an impact on relationships with other loved ones and friends. It is common for caregivers to feel that no one understands what they are going through and that dealing with the challenges is a lonely experience.

How do you know when you are stressed? Are you...

- feeling irritable and impatient with others?

- unable to sleep through the night?

- experiencing a change in appetite?

- unable to laugh and have a good time?

- having difficulty keeping your mind on something?

- having no interest in your own appearance or cleanliness?

- withdrawing from or avoiding other people?

How can you manage stress?

- Managing stress is a continual process. Before you can start managing your stress, you first have to understand what causes you to experience stress and how you react to it in particular situations. Also, think about what coping strategies work for you. Once you identify these factors, you can start managing stress and effectively using stress reduction techniques, such as those that mentioned below.

- Stress reduction techniques can help provide relief from stress when it occurs as well as help prevent stress from building up. They are proven methods of dealing with stress and can have a positive effect on your health, since relieving stress reduces the risk of developing health problems.

How can you prevent stress?

- Take time out for yourself in order to stay connected with others and to provide you necessary breaks from caregiving, even if it is just 15 minutes at a time.

SECTION
6

- Take a walk or make time for other physical exercise and healthy physical outlets.

- Make time to spend with friends and family you enjoy.

- Call friends, neighbors or family on the phone to stay in touch with others.

- It's still important to laugh! Remember and use your sense of humor. Listen to tapes, records, television or people that help you laugh.

- Talk things out with a friend or get professional counseling if needed.

- Learn and practice relaxation techniques.

- Maintain religious or spiritual practices that are important to you (e.g., attend church or synagogue, pray, read religious literature).

- Ask for additional help from others. This might be support from a family member, neighbor, or from a paid service. Formal support might include hiring someone for a few hours to stay with the person you care for, or having them attend an adult day center.

- Engage in pleasant activities, even small ones, in order to help feel more relaxed and happy.

  - Watch your favorite television show.

  - Buy yourself flowers.

  - Go out to dinner or a movie.

  - Pleasant events can also involve the person with dementia, such as looking at photos together or singing hymns together at church.

  - Try to solve problems as they come up, rather than avoiding them. Ask for help or let others help you.

  - Establish priorities and organize time more effectively. Let the small stuff go. Again, ask for help or let others help you.

  - Try to stop running negative thoughts and attitudes through your mind, and learn healthier ways of thinking about yourself and your situation.

  - Take time for your physical health.

  - Keep your own doctor, dentist and other professional healthcare appointments.

  - Take prescribed medications as suggested by your health care professional.

  - Try to get enough sleep and rest. Talk with your healthcare professional and other caregivers about ways to get enough rest.

  - Avoid smoking or relying on alcohol or drugs to feel better.

How can you relieve stress when it occurs?

When caring for a family member who has dementia, you might find yourself in situations that are very distressing and upsetting. The following "stress reduction techniques" will decrease your stress when you are dealing with a stressful situation. These techniques can also be used throughout the day before stressful situations occur so that you feel more relaxed and focused.

Deep Breathing

- Taking a deep breath helps to relax your muscles. To do this, take a deep breath in and hold it for a few seconds; usually 3 or 4 seconds is long enough. Do not breathe so deeply or so long that it becomes uncomfortable. As you exhale, try to relax the muscles in your jaw, shoulders and arms, letting them go loose and limp. Try taking several deep breaths in a row to get added stress relief. Another option while doing this exercise is to say a word to yourself such as "relax," "peace," or "let go" while you are exhaling.

Counting Exercise

- To do this, take a deep breath in. Slowly let the air out, counting either from 1 to 10 or from 10 to 1.

Listening to Music

- Purposely playing a favorite song or a favorite type of music can be very relaxing.

Visual Imagery Exercise

- Picturing a relaxing image in your head can have a relaxing physical effect on your body. Try this by closing your eyes and imagining a relaxing object, place or activity. One example may be walking on a quiet beach at sunset. Imagine the sound of the waves gently rolling onto shore, the smell of the sea salt air, the feel of warm sand underneath your feet, and the sight of the setting sun creating beautiful colors in the sky. Perhaps you collect a couple of interesting shells or watch a sea gull walk in and out of the waves. You can experiment with the details of your visual imagery, adding to it or changing it to create a scenario that is most relaxing for you.

Progressive Muscle Relaxation

- Muscle relaxation can help to relieve physical tension in your body's muscles as a result of stress. This exercise can be beneficial, but should not be done if you have any pain, injury to your joints, or any other condition where strenuous activity is not advised. Begin by bending your arm at your elbow to "make a muscle." Squeeze the muscle very tightly and hold for three seconds. Then relax. Continue by making a fist. Squeeze your fist very tightly and hold for three seconds. Then relax. Straighten your arm and let it hang loose by your side. Think about the contrast in feeling when your muscles are tense and when they are relaxed. This progressive muscle relaxation exercise is a way to work toward decreasing muscle tension and tightness. These are only a few stress reduction techniques that might be helpful for you. It is important to try different techniques to see which one works best for you. It is also important to keep practicing these techniques. The more you use them, the more effective they will be in helping relieve stress. Also, try to keep a record of the situations you find most stressful and how the different stress reduction techniques work for you in these situations. Use the "Stress Diary" provided in Section 8 of this guide.

SECTION
6

The information presented here on stress has been adapted from the NIH REACH I and II Study Materials: Belle et al., Enhancing the Quality of Life of Dementia Caregivers from Different Ethnic or Racial Groups: A Randomized, Controlled Trial. *Annals of Internal Medicine* 145(10): 727-738; Gitlin, L.N., et al. (2003). Effect of multi-component interventions on caregiver burden and depression: The REACH multi-site initiative at six months follow-up. *Psychology and Aging* 18(3): 361-374.

SECTION

6

Strategies for Specific Behaviors

Agitation

What Is Agitation?

Agitation is considered a syndrome of behaviors that may include excessive motor behaviors, aggressiveness, restlessness, or distress. Agitation may not be an obvious expression of need or confusion. The most commonly observed behaviors of this syndrome are restlessness, pacing, complaining, repetitive sentences, negativity and requests for attention, cursing, and verbal or physical aggression. Agitation occurs in most people diagnosed with dementia at some stage of their illness.

- *Mild agitation* refers to behaviors that are somewhat disruptive to others, but are non-aggressive and pose little risk of danger. Caregivers can feel stressed by the frequency of the behaviors and constant need for redirection. Examples of mild agitation include moaning, crying, arguing, pacing, speaking inappropriately to strangers, asking repetitive questions, making repetitive movements, using the telephone inappropriately, wandering, or constant movement around the home.

- *Severe agitation* may produce aggressive behavior that is very disruptive and/or poses a threat of physical harm to self or others. Efforts to set limits and redirect the person with dementia are generally ineffective. Examples of severe agitation include screaming, insisting on trying to leave the home or getting lost in public places, making feeding difficult, throwing objects, grabbing and scratching caregivers, head-banging or injuring oneself.

Why Might Agitation Occur?

It is important to identify what may be causing a person's agitation. It may be that the person has an unmet need that they are unable to communicate clearly or there may be conditions in the environment that prompt agitated behaviors.

Common Triggers

Possible Health Factors

- Pain or physical illness
- Urinary retention
- Constipation or fecal impaction
- Dehydration
- Fatigue/tiredness
- Hallucinations or delusions
- Loss of control of behaviors due to the physical changes to the brain
- Delirium
- Side effect of a medication
- Depression or Anxiety

Defensive Behavior

- Impatience or irritation on the part of others in the household
- Activities requiring close personal contact, such as toileting, bathing, or dressing
- Rushed or hurried activities
- Challenges or corrections to the person's beliefs or delusions
- Invasion of personal space or possessions

Feelings of Failure

- Arguments, contradictions, or scolding by another person
- A sense of rejection
- Capabilities are being overtaxed — being asked to do too much; expectations of them are too high

Feelings of Fear

- Feelings of insecurity, anger, fear or frustration
- Perceived threat
- Strangers
- Isolation

Need for Attention

- Unmet needs such as hunger, thirst, boredom or a full bladder

Possible Environmental Factors

- Change in location, including vacations or hospitalization
- Distortion of light, dark, time, space or sleep cycles
- Over-stimulation (e.g., too much noise or too many people)
- Change in routine
- Lack of structure
- Social isolation

SECTION

7

Strategies for Preventing Agitation

- Ignore the person with dementia's mistakes.

- Avoid over-stimulation by simplifying and de-cluttering the home environment.

- Create a quiet uncluttered place for the person with dementia if he/she becomes very emotional.

- Eliminate questions/comments that are abstract or require abstract thought or that you do not think that the person with dementia will be able to respond to.

- Be aware of the warning signs of agitation.

- Reduce stimulus such as turning off radios and televisions.

- Schedule regular rest breaks.

- Eliminate glare from lighting.

- Avoid use of caffeine.

- Ensure that there is an unrushed and consistent routine.

- Set up a structured routine that includes activities that match the person's interest and abilities.

What to Do If the Person with Dementia Becomes Upset

- Explain what is happening step-by-step, in simple sentences using a calm tone.

- Even if the person with dementia cannot understand your words, your calm tones may be reassuring.

- Consult the person with dementia's doctor and/or a psychiatrist.

- This will help determine if there are any physical or mental health concerns that are causing or worsening the agitation.

- Be calm and positive in your manner when you talk with the person you are caring for.

- The emotions you or others convey when you talk to the person you are caring for may influence his or her response. The person you care for will sense negative feelings like anger or frustration in your manner, and this can trigger a negative response. Use low tones and a slow rate of speech.

- Engage the person you care for in constructive activities. These may help to reduce restlessness. Simple repetitive tasks like folding laundry or stirring soup may be helpful.

- Engage the person you care for in pleasant events.

- A simple activity such as having a cup of tea or looking at old photographs together might calm down the person you care for.

- Safeguard the environment.

- Make sure the person you care for cannot accidentally injure him/herself with things he/she may get into, especially in the kitchen (stove, knives) or bathroom (cleaning solutions, medications). Also make sure he/she cannot get out of the house and wander away.

- Play along with the beliefs of the person you care for.

- Play calming music.

- Introduce a form of physical activity or exercise.

- Lower your expectations and demands. Try to reduce demands while still enabling the person you care for to feel worthwhile through their contributions (such as folding towels instead of doing laundry). Try not to put the person you care for in a failure-oriented situation.

- Reassure the person you care for that everything will be ok, using a calm tone of voice.

- Allow pacing if the person you care for is not harming him/herself or anyone else.

- Be supportive and encouraging.

- Distract or re-direct the person you care for to another activity if he or she starts to get agitated. For example, you could ask the person you care for to fold laundry or watch a favorite television show.

Repeating Questions

What Are Repetitive Questions?

Repetitive questioning refers to the constant repeating of a question throughout the day. Common questions asked repeatedly might include *"What day is it?"* *"What time is it?"* and *"Am I going to the Adult Day Center tomorrow?"* These questions can be very bothersome to family members. These types of questions can be very irritating or upsetting to caregivers.

Why Might Repetitive Questions Occur?

While repetitive questions occur for a variety of reasons, oftentimes it is because something is bothering the person with dementia, but they can't remember what the answer is. The answer they received is quickly forgotten but the question is not.

Common Triggers

- The inability to remember that the same question was already asked
- Inability to judge time (or knowing how long the caregiver has been away)
- Anxiety about what is happening or might happen in the near future
- Feeling a loss of control
- Fear of separation from the caregiver
- Seeking attention
- Side effects from medication
- Misinterpretation of sounds or noises
- Inability to express needs (hunger, need to go to the toilet)

Strategies

- Pay attention to what you say to the person with dementia and what he/she repeats.

- For example, let's say you tell the person with dementia about an event that will occur later in the day or that you will be taking him/her out to see the doctor. If he/she then repeatedly asks *"When are we leaving?"* then it may be more helpful not to inform the person with dementia too far in advance of the actual event.

- Respond to the emotion behind what the person with dementia is saying. When the person with dementia repeats a question over and over, such as *"What am I doing today?"* it may mean that he/she is feeling lost and uncertain or frightened. A response to this feeling may help to reassure him/her.

- Give the person with dementia a hug or a pat on the arm.

- Use reassuring tones.

- Use reassuring words such as, *"You are always safe here with me."*

- Give your full attention.

- Create a memory board for the areas of the house in which the person with dementia spends the most time. Memory boards, such as a dry-erase board, can help the person with dementia remember and access basic information. Memory boards are a good tool to use with repetitive questions involving time/place/person, phone numbers and activities/events. They can be hung or placed wherever the person with dementia is most likely to easily see or find them. If he/she is asking a question that can be answered by looking at the board, you can remind him/her to look there.

- Create index cards. When the person with dementia repeatedly asks questions, the question and answer can be written on an index card that he/she keeps on or near at all times. This card can be kept in a shirt, coat or pants pocket, or in a wallet or purse. For example, write the answer to a question, such as *"What time is dinner?"* on the card; refer the person with dementia to the card when answering.

- Refer to a calendar. Forgetting or not knowing the date and day of the week are common problems for people with memory problems. This symptom of memory loss will not improve, but you can learn ways to cope with it, such as referring the person with dementia to a calendar.

  - One example of a calendar you could buy is a page-a-day calendar.

  - Make sure that the words and numbers on the calendar are large enough that the person with dementia can easily see them.

  - Place the calendar near where she sits or lays.

  - Refer to the calendar every day. This is so that the person with dementia gets into the habit of referring to it.

- Divert the person with dementia to another activity, instead of reminding him or her that they have already asked the question; for instance, try distracting with a walk, food or favorite activity.

- Try to keep the routines of the person you are caring for as consistent as possible, especially during the times that he/she is most likely to repeat questions.

- Use a calm voice when responding to repeated questions.

- Remove the cause of the repetitive question.

- If an object such as a mirror, a car, a coat, a television remote control or a picture seems to trigger the question, try to hide the object.

- Seek additional services to aid you in caring for the person with dementia.

- If you still feel overwhelmed by these repetitive questions after trying these strategies, it may be time to seek additional help. This could include other family members or friends, adult day centers, in-home respite services, or home health aides.

Inappropriate Screaming, Crying Out, or Other Disruptive Sounds

What Are Inappropriate Sounds?

These are vocal behaviors that may be disturbing to others. The meaning of these vocalizations or their significance may be unclear. The noises might be intermittent or continuous, with or without purpose, and varying in level of loudness. These inappropriate sounds may include screaming, nonsensical verbal noises, talking incoherently, repeating the same word over and over, moaning, swearing or whistling.

Why Might Inappropriate Sounds Occur?

Brain damage caused by the dementia can cause this type of behavior, usually in the advanced stage of the dementia.

Common Triggers

- Inability to express other needs such as hunger, thirst, fatigue, or needing to use the bathroom
- Pain or discomfort
- Too much noise or stimulation in the room
- The behavior of others in the room
- Frustration because there is not enough stimulation in the room
- Feeling there is a lack of meaning or purpose, or boredom
- Anxiety about what is happening
- Feeling a loss of control
- Needing one-on-one attention
- Lowered inhibitions
- Depression, loneliness or anxiety
- Isolation

Strategies

- Limit the number of choices the person with dementia is given.

- Encourage family and friends to spend more time with the person with dementia
  The person with dementia may be lonely and trying to connect with someone.
  If you think the person with dementia is trying to get your attention, try having people spend more one-on-one time with them. This could include time spent giving your family member a manicure, reading to them, brushing their hair, or just talking to them.

- Identify activities or circumstances that help to calm the person you are caring for.
  - Play soothing music.
  - Have the person you are caring for sit in a favorite room or by a favorite window.
  - Talk to the person you are caring for in a soothing, calm voice.
  - Use a consistent, predictable routine.
  - Use the past hobbies and interests of the person you are caring for to develop simple activities that he or she might be interested in.

- Give the person you are caring for special attention when he or she is not shouting or screaming.

- Make sure the person you are caring for is wearing his/her glasses and hearing aids.

- Speak with the doctor about the behavior.
  - The screaming may be related to an underlying depression and may improve with treatment with an antidepressant.
  - Have the doctor check for urinary tract infection, sinus infection, abdominal pain, or adverse effects of a medication.

Constant Arguing or Complaining

What Is Constant Arguing or Complaining?

This includes arguments or complaints that are made either constantly throughout the day or at one time during the day about a particular subject. For example, arguments might be made daily when it is time to get dressed or bathed. Ongoing complaints might be made about going to an adult day center.

Why Might Constant Arguing or Complaining Occur?

Try to identify the source or trigger of the arguments or complaints. For example, the person with dementia might argue or complain about attending an adult day center or going to bed at night. Refer to the *"Six Steps to Managing Behaviors"* at the beginning of this guide to come up with strategies that might make these situations more agreeable to the person with dementia.

Common Triggers

- Anxiety about what is happening
- Feeling a loss of control
- Fear of separation from the caregiver
- Need for attention
- Lack of inhibition due to changes in the brain
- Personality changes due to changes in the brain

Strategies

- Identify activities or circumstances that help keep the person with dementia calm.
- Play soothing music.
- Have the person with dementia sit in a favorite room or by a favorite window.
- Talk to the person with dementia in a soothing, calm voice.

- Use a consistent, predictable routine.

- Use the person with dementias past hobbies and interests to develop simple activities that he or she might enjoy.

- Acknowledge and validate the emotions behind what the person with dementia is saying.

- Distract or re-direct the person with dementia to another activity if he or she starts to argue or complain.

  - For example, you could ask the person with dementia to come help you wash some lettuce in the kitchen or watch a favorite old movie.

- Support your position/argument using the words of an authority figure, such as a doctor. There are some situations for which the person with dementia may be more likely to listen to or believe someone else. For instance, the person with dementia might argue less about not being able to drive or about having to attend an adult day service if they think it is because the doctor ordered it.

- Avoid responding to the person with dementia's constant complaints or long-standing arguments. If there is an argument or complaint that the person with dementia has made frequently in the past, try not responding to it or walking away. This will help avoid making the situation worse.

- Use music to avoid listening to the arguments and complaints. Some caregivers find that using a Walkman allows them to stay in the same room or area as their family member and still be able to relax.

- Speak with the doctor about the behavior; the arguing or complaining may be related to an underlying depression and may improve with treatment such as an antidepressant.

Wandering

What Is Wandering?

There are many definitions of wandering. Wandering can be considered simply as a form of aimless walking or walking in search of someone or something that is not realistic or attainable. Wandering may also involve excessive moving around either during the day or at night. Wandering becomes most dangerous when it involves attempts to leave home either through a door or window.

"Sundowning" is a form of wandering that refers to pacing in the late afternoon or early evening. "Shadowing" is a form of wandering as well. It refers to when a person closely follows and often imitates the actions of another person.

In this section you will find strategies related to wandering inside the home, including strategies related to changing daily routines and the home environment, wandering at night, shadowing, and wandering outside.

Why Might Wandering Occur?

The best approach to minimizing wandering will depend on the specific reason why the behavior occurs. It is important to determine if the wandering is dangerous to the person and if the behavior can be allowed to continue.

While the causes of sundowning are not well understood, possible explanations include biochemical factors, sensory overload or deprivation, and stress, isolation or fear. Dehydration and low light levels are thought to add to sundowning.

Common Triggers

- In search of someone or something familiar for security
- May have had a work role that involved walking
- May start wandering at a time in the day when he/she either had walked to work, walked to lunch or home, or walked to visit with friends
- Searching for someone in the family (deceased spouse or child)
- Walking may have been a favored form of stress reduction or exercise
- Frustration and trying to leave a particular situation
- Boredom
- Anxiety
- Not knowing where he/she is
- May have a physical need, such as hunger or the need to use the toilet
- Broken sleep patterns may cause restlessness and disorientation in the middle of the night
- Effect of a medication
- Confusion about what time it is

Strategies

Changes to Home

- Provide opportunities for safe wandering in the home.
- Use childproof latches on kitchen cabinets, appliances, and any place where cleaning supplies or other chemicals are kept.
- Secure handrails, broken steps, and loose carpeting in key rooms, on stairs and in hallways.
- Use an electronic monitor (such as the kind used to monitor babies) to supervise activities from another room.
- Install bells or alarms on doors, cabinets or drawers that can alert you when they are opened.

SECTION

7

- Install an automatic shut-off switch on the stove to prevent burns or fire.

- Install a shut-off switch on electrical or gas lines.

- Because the person with dementia's depth perception may be impaired, also consider these other strategies to enhance safe wandering in the home, particularly in stairways and hallways:

  - Paint a narrow strip of contrasting color at the edge of each step or use colored tape.

  - Paint the wall in the stairwell a contrasting color from the steps in order to accentuate the stair rise.

  - Adjust the lighting to provide even illumination without shadows or pools of bright light.

  - Install window coverings to eliminate glare in key rooms and passageways throughout the house.

  - At night, use two or three dim sources of light in the bedroom to eliminate shadows. Shadows can be mistaken for many things and make the person with dementia fearful. However, be careful not to over-illuminate the bedroom and risk waking your family member.

- Encourage the person with dementia to use a stable rocking chair that can also be used when he/she is restless.

- Provide tactile stimulation:

  - Introduce interesting things to touch such as a touchstone, three-dimensional wall arts or an activity board.

  - Keep objects to touch accessible and in full view of the person with dementia.

- Provide visual stimulation:

  - Introduce a book of meaningful photos.

  - Have magazines accessible that may be of interest.

  - Remove or hide unnecessary objects.

- Use a screen or curtain to hide distracting items from view. A simple home environment is less distracting and may not invite the person with dementia to look for lost objects.

- Create a low-stimulus setting for periodic rest breaks for the person with dementia. Play pleasing music, such as nature sounds.

- If the person with dementia is looking for lost or misplaced items, purchase duplicates (keys, wallets, etc.) and produce these items when necessary.

- Alternatively, an old key can be used to replace the real car keys, which are kept out of sight.

Changes to Daily Routines

- Provide safe outlets for wandering.

- Consider opportunities for regular outlets for walking such as visiting a museum, mall-walking, and strolling around the neighborhood or yard.

- Use redirection. This could include having the person walk over to a table to participate in an activity, or simply turning the person away from a door or a particular area.

- Use distraction. Provide some work or leisure outlet. This is especially useful during times of the day when wandering typically happens, such as in the early evening. Develop a work-like routine to perform at sundown (such as putting way all papers kept on a desk.

- Increase opportunities for exercise during the day.
  - Consider using basic exercise equipment.
  - Ask for or purchase help from a friend or neighbor to take the person with dementia out for a walk every day.

- Consider enrolling the person in an adult day care that can provide supervised and structured activity.

- Be objective.
  - Try not to take the person with dementia's wandering personally. He or she is probably trying to make sense of a world that no longer seems predictable.
  - Talk to the person with dementia's doctor about possible anxiety or depression that may be contributing to the wandering.

Strategies for Wandering at Night

- Limit the number of naps during the day.
  - If people have too much rest during the day, it may be hard for them to fall asleep at night. Have activities or tasks available to help keep the person you are caring for awake.
  - Provide appropriate physical activity and exercise each day.
  - Provide plenty of exposure to bright light, either natural or artificial, ideally in the early morning. This will help you set the person with dementia's internal clock.
  - Avoid liquids containing caffeine for a couple of hours before bedtime. Remember that tea, many soft drinks and coffee contain caffeine. Sugar and chocolate also can keep a person from sleeping.
  - Avoid heavy meals with meats, such as beef or pork, thick sauces, or rich desserts right before bedtime.

SECTION
7

- Establish a routine before bed that prepares the person with dementia for sleep.
  - Choose activities that are soothing and pleasant, but not exciting. Try a backrub, warm bath or soft music to reduce anxiety and promote relaxation.
  - Set up a regular sleeping time.
  - Try to have the person with dementia get ready for bed at the same time each night so that he or she will come to expect it as part of the daily routine.
  - Make sure that the person with dementia uses the bathroom immediately prior to going to bed. Try these other strategies if the person with dementia frequently needs to urinate in the middle of the night:
  - The person with dementia may wake up at night because of the need to use the bathroom. It may be easier for the person with dementia to have a commode or a urinal close to the bed at night so that they do not have to go all the way to the bathroom.

- Individuals who cannot control urinating sometimes wake up at night because of wetness. Incontinence underwear, such as Depends, might help reduce the discomfort of wetness.

- If the person with dementia wakes during the night, orient and reassure him/her by saying something like, *"Everything is fine; it is not time to be awake yet; please go back to sleep."*

- Keep explanations to a minimum; redirect with *"It's nighttime; let's go back to sleep."*

- Keep the bedroom at a comfortable temperature.

- Keep the bedroom quiet.

- Use the bedroom for sleeping and not for other activities.

- Talk with the person with dementia's doctor.

- It may be possible to change time or dosage of medications that might be keeping the person with dementia awake at night, or to add a medication that will help the person with dementia sleep more restfully at night. Some people, for example those with back problems or arthritis, may wake up because of pain.

Strategies for Shadowing

- Reassure the person with dementia that you are not going anywhere.

- Remember that the person with dementia might be shadowing you due to confusion or anxiety. Providing reassurance will help lessen these feelings.

- Sing or hum or talk while in the next room so that the person with dementia can hear that you are close by.

- Provide the person with dementia with an activity to do. This will help direct the person with dementia's attention to something other than following you.

- If the person with dementia is unwilling to do an activity on their own, such as watching television, then try engaging them in part of the task you are doing. For instance, the person with dementia could help set the table or fold the laundry.

- Avoid talking about leaving or plans to leave; this will keep the person with dementia from becoming anxious that you are leaving.

Strategies for Wandering Outside the Home

- Install or change the lock on outside doors.

- Consider a keyed deadbolt or an additional lock positioned high or low on the door (out of reach of the person with dementia).

- Place a large "Stop" sign or "Employees Only" sign on doors that lead outside.

- Place bells or alarms on doors to alert you when they are opened.

- Place a door mat that plays music when you step on it. This may distract the person with dementia.

- Use fabric, curtain or wallpaper to disguise the door.

- Use fabric or other material to cover the doorknob, locks or windows.

- Place a note on the door that says "Stay Home."

- Keep entrance area dark.

- Install motion sensor lights outside.

- Fence in the backyard, this will allow the person with dementia to be outside safely

- Place locks on fence gates.

- Be prepared for other types of wandering. Individuals with dementia have been known to drive for very long distances either in their own car or in someone else's. You can prevent these problems by keeping car keys out of sight or by temporarily disabling the car by removing its distributor cap.

How to Keep a Person Safe If Wandering Outside Occurs

- Enroll in the Alzheimer's Association Safe Return Program, a nationwide identification system designed to assist in the safe return of people who become lost when wandering. You can do this by contacting the Alzheimer's Association.

- Use a Medic Alert bracelet or keep a card with name and address in the pocket of the person with dementia. The bracelet is available through the Alzheimer's Association.

- Keep a recent photograph or videotape of the person with dementia. This will assist police if he or she becomes lost.

- Inform neighbors and other local community members and businesses. Individuals in your local community can be on the lookout for the person you are caring for and can call you if they suspect he or she is wandering or can help with a safe return.

SECTION
7

- Keep a list of neighbor's names and phone numbers easily accessible.

- Teach neighbors how to approach the person with dementia if they are assisting them in returning home:
  - Approach the person from the front.
  - Introduce yourself.
  - Offer help and reestablish the day, date and time.
  - Avoid pulling or pushing the person.

- Keep a list of emergency phone numbers and addresses of the local police and fire departments and hospitals, as well as the Safe Return help line easily accessible (e.g., on refrigerator).

- Keep an up to date list of medications that is easily accessible in case emergency medical personnel need this information.

Restlessness or Constant Motion

What Is Restlessness or Constant Motion?

Restlessness is closely associated with agitation, a common problem in dementing illnesses such as Alzheimer's disease. For instance, sometimes individuals with dementia who are agitated become restless and start pacing or fidgeting. One form of restlessness is called "sundowning." Sundowning behavior is defined as a restlessness or agitation that may begin in the late afternoon. Individuals who experience sundowning may become more agitated or confused in the afternoon and evening. Sundowning can be a very troublesome behavior and exhausting to family caregivers.

Why Might Restlessness Occur?

Try to identify the time of day, situations or events that trigger restlessness. Such "triggers" may be aspects of the environment or interactions with people that never used to bother the person with dementia.

Common Triggers

- Underlying medical condition causing pain and discomfort
- Anxiety
- Worry about lost or misplaced items
- Unfamiliar environment
- Looking for someone or something, such as "home"
- Feeling worried or lost
- Boredom

Strategies

- Schedule daily activities in the morning and simple, calming activities in the afternoon if the person with dementia is restless.

- Avoid caffeine use.

- Avoid over-stimulation by simplifying and de-cluttering the home environment. Create a quiet uncluttered place for the person with dementia if he/she becomes very restless.

- Engage the person you care for in other activities. These may help to reduce restlessness by giving him/her something to focus on. Simple repetitive tasks like folding laundry or stirring soup may be helpful. A simple activity as having a cup of tea or looking at old photographs together might also help.

- Play soothing or calming music.

- Consider pacing to be a positive form of physical exercise.

- Plan to spend time with the person you care for when he or she is most likely to become restless.

- Explain what is happening step-by-step in simple sentences. Even if the person you care for cannot understand your words, your calm tones can be reassuring.

- Consult the doctor of the person you care for. A medical examination will help identify any physical problems, psychotic symptoms, anxiety or depression, or side effects of medication.

- Safeguard the environment.
  - Make sure the person you care for cannot accidentally injure him/herself with things he/she may get into, especially in the kitchen (stove, knives) or bathroom (cleaning solutions, medications).

- Make sure he/she cannot get out of the house and wander away.

Rummaging and Hoarding

What Are Rummaging and Hoarding Behaviors?

Rummaging involves going through one's own or another's belongings or other items in closets, kitchen drawers or dressers. The objective of the search may not even exist, may be something from the past, or the search could be legitimate. In some cases, the person with dementia may take a dresser or bureau completely apart. A related behavior is hoarding, taking items and hiding them. Hoarding can pose a health hazard when perishable foods are hoarded.

Why Might Rummaging and Hoarding Occur?

Look for possible causes for the behavior. Rummaging may be an outlet for agitation. Hoarding sometimes occurs when people believe others are taking their belongings.

Common Triggers for Rummaging

- Seeking tactile/sensory stimulation
- Boredom
- Trying to find an object of interest
- Wanting to feel productive

Common Triggers for Hoarding

- Trying to gain a sense of control
- Responding to a lifelong pattern of saving things, such as a person who lived through the Great Depression
- Trying to hold on to something in light of the losses he/she is experiencing

Strategies

Changes to the Home Environment

Consider giving the person with dementia an interesting and safe place to rummage, in an area or room that you will not mind becoming cluttered.

- Set up a chest of drawers, plastic containers or boxes filled with different objects.
- Set up a desk with office material that you family member can use.
- Set up a photo gallery in which the person with dementia can rearrange the photos.
- Give the person with dementia safe objects to hoard such as a napkin or old keys.
- Keep magazines or coffee table books available to be picked up or looked at.
- Place small objects such as costume jewelry or beads in a container for the person with dementia to sort, put in, and take out.
- Highlight a drawer or area for rummaging with color duct tape or paint.
- Fill a top drawer with things that can be rummaged through.
- Provide objects for sorting such as laundry, utensils, beads and money.

Increase opportunities for sensory stimulation:

- Introduce pleasant music.

- Introduce tactile (touch) experiences such as playing with clay or cooking.

- Create a sensory stimulation board or a handyman's box containing such items as latches, knobs and locks.

Remove objects to minimize possible damage from rummaging and hoarding:

- If the person with dementia hides objects and then looks for them, provide him/her with a special place where items can be kept safely.

- Place valuables such as keys out of sight and reach.

- Keep perishable and opened foods out of sight.

- Use childproof locks on refrigerator or kitchen cabinets.

- Remove valuable glass objects.

- Disguise or camouflage doorknobs and door handles by painting them the same color as the background.

- Place a sign that says "NO!" on places you want the person with dementia to stay out of.

Changes to Daily Routine

Establish a daily routine that includes exercise and meaningful activities.

- Introduce productive activities. Have the person with dementia wash a window, use a vacuum cleaner, wash dishes, or fold towels (e.g., activities that use large motor and repetitive motions).

- Look for patterns. If the person with dementia keeps taking the same object, such as a watch or a pair of glasses, give him or her an inexpensive one of their own to keep.

- Keep everyday items in view. This way the person with dementia will not need to look for them.

Refusing or Resisting Care

What Does It Mean to Refuse or Reject Care?

Refusing or rejecting care may take various forms. A person with dementia may become agitated and resist help with daily activities by pulling away or leaving the area, crying or loud exclamations, verbal and physical aggression such as cursing, biting, grabbing, pushing, or threatening.

SECTION
7

In this section you will first find general strategies related to changes to the home environment and to daily routines that will make the completion of daily activities easier both for you and the person with dementia. Following this general information you will find information specific to bathing, dressing, eating and grooming.

Why Might a Person with Dementia Refuse or Reject Care?

Resistance usually occurs during hands-on care involving bathing, dressing, toileting, eating, administering medication, or going to the doctor's office. The person may not understand what the care is for and why it is important. He or she may find it bothersome.

Common Triggers

- Fear, pain or distress
- Confusion as to what to do
- Discomfort
- Loss of control
- Over-stimulation or too many distractions
- Self-protective behavior
- Inability to recognize or understand caregiver's actions
- Invasion of personal space
- Expression of an unmet or unidentified need

General Strategies

Changes to the Home Environment

- Warm the room sufficiently so that an activity, such as removing clothing, is comfortable for the person with dementia.

- Set out only the items that are needed for the activity.

- Arrange items in the order they will be used. For example, place grooming supplies out in the order in which they are needed.

- Write 2- to 3-step directions on a large poster board. If reading is a problem, use pictures or drawings.

- Place objects within the field of vision of the person with dementia, so that he or she will be more likely to find it.

- Eliminate objects that are not necessary for that activity, such as extra dishes or newspapers on the kitchen table, so that the objects will not distract or confuse the person with dementia.

- Use an electronic monitoring device to supervise activities from another room.

- Modify doorways to make the room easier to enter by widening, opening or lowering thresholds.

- Use a screen or curtain to hide distracting items.

- Keep an object available that can serve as a distraction to the person with dementia if he or she begins to behave problematically.

- Eliminate unpleasant or harmful odors such as urine and cleaning fluids.

- Keep background noise such as TV and radio low so that they do not distract the person with dementia.

- Encourage use of eyeglasses and dentures.

- Use a safety gate in doorways to keep the person with dementia in or out of certain rooms such as the bathroom or a stairway. This gate should be tall enough so that the person with dementia will see it and not stumble over it. Do not use a safety gate at the top of stairs as this is a hazard for falls and injury.

- Use bells or alarms placed on doors, cabinet doors or drawers that can alert you if they are opened.

- Use a lock or safety latches on cabinets, drawers and/or doors.

- Adjust lighting. Use window covering or shears to eliminate glare. Place more lights in a room in order to get rid of shadows.

- Keep all stairways and passageways free of objects.

Changes to the Daily Routine

- If the person with dementia does something in an unusual but effective way, do not correct him or her. Ignore mistakes that are of no significance, such as clothing that clashes.

- Establish a calm and accepting atmosphere when helping the person with dementia carry out daily care activities.

- One important reason for offering positive encouragement is that many people with dementia may be sensitive to caregivers' emotions. If the person with dementia senses that you are upset or frustrated, he or she is likely to become even more upset or frustrated.

- Allow the person with dementia as much time as needed to complete a task.

- Establish routines around each of the care activities, such as going to bed at the same time every day or taking the person with dementia to the bathroom after each meal.

SECTION
7

- Use different ways to show the person with dementia what to do:
  - Demonstrate the action you want the person with dementia to do.
  - Use simple, clear, one-step directions, such as *"Put soap on the washcloth"* or *"Open your mouth."*
  - Use hand-over-hand guiding to help the person with dementia complete the activity.

- Help with the activity only as much as is really necessary.

- If the person with dementia is unable to wash his/her feet, help with this part of bathing only and merely supervise the remainder of the other steps involved in bathing.

- Ask yourself, "Is it really necessary that I do this task or that this task is done in this way? Can it be done later or by someone else?"

- Expand your support network to include paid and unpaid help who will provide assistance with tasks such as bathing, dressing, and/or feeding/eating.

- Make a schedule of daily helpers and their specific jobs.

- Teach others how to do the specific routine.

- Ask your doctor or pharmacist about the possible side effects of medications on the individual's ability to participate in daily care activities.

Strategies to Manage Resistance to Bathing

Changes to the Bathtub

- Put a few drops of blue food coloring in the tub water to make the water easier to see. This may also make the tub water appear more inviting.

- Use a thermometer to check the water temperature. Pay attention to complaints of being too hot or cold.

- Set the temperature on the hot water heater so that it does not exceed 120° F.

- Use tub chair/bench or hand-held shower hose for bathing.

- Place colored tape around edge of tub to increase contrast.

- Install grab bars in the bathtub.

- Remove glass shower doors on bathtubs or alter bathing area for easier access.

SECTION
7

Changes to the Bathroom

- Use brightly colored items for bathing (soap, soap dish, towels).

- Paint the door to the bathroom a bright, eye-catching color.

- Remove locks on the bathroom door or change its location.

- Place a non-skid mat on floor of bathroom

Introduce sensory stimulation to relax the person with dementia.

- Use aromas to make the bathing experience pleasant.
- Use soft, relaxing music.

Changes to the Bathing Routine

- Hand each bathing item to the person with dementia one at a time as they are to be used.
- Provide a large, warm towel or blanket after the bath. This will help keep the person with dementia warm after bathing. A towel can also be used during bathing to cover private areas and will also help maintain privacy.
- Use a hand-held shower when bathing the person with dementia if he or she seems frightened by the water.
- Establish a calm and reassuring atmosphere when bathing, especially when the person with dementia is getting into and out of the tub or shower.
- Avoid scolding, criticizing or invading the personal space of the person with dementia, especially if he/she shows signs of being agitated.
- Do not talk to the person with dementia if he or she needs to concentrate on walking to the bathroom or when getting into and out of the tub/shower.
- Compliment the person with dementia about how clean he/she is and the amount of effort demonstrated.
- Allow adequate time for the person with dementia to adjust to changes in light intensity.
- Provide a safe place to stand or sit until eyes accommodate to the difference.
- Consider alternate bathing schedules. For example, consider a semi-weekly tub bath or daily sponge baths.
- Try bathing the person with dementia in the morning when he or she is well rested.

Strategies to Manage Resistance to Dressing

Changes to the Home Environment

- Remove from closet all out-of-season, ill-fitting, or little-used clothing.
- Arrange closets and drawers so that like items are kept together.
- Use clothing that is easy to put on and take off. For example, Velcro closures, pull-on clothing and elastic waistbands are simple to handle.
- Use shoes with elastic laces or with Velcro closures.
- Install countertop, shelving, a closet organizer or extra space to arrange clothing.

Changes to the Dressing Routine

- Limit choice about styles and colors.

- Lay out the clothes in the order the person with dementia will put them on.

- Purchase items that can be mixed and matched in different ways.
  - One suggestion is to choose a few basic colors and buy all solid trousers/shirts in those colors.
  - Blouses/sweaters/shirts can also be purchased within the selected color scheme and may be either print or solid fabrics.
  - Put a package together of one set of clothing.
  - A package of clothing could include underwear, socks, etc. In this way, you can hand the person with dementia the package and they will not have to search for these items.

- Establish one place in the bedroom where all clothing needed for the morning can be found.

- Remove dirty clothes from the room on a routine basis so that the person with dementia will not put them on again.

- Hand each item of clothing to the person with dementia one at a time as they are to be put on.

- Use simple, clear, one-step directions, such as *"Put your arm in your sleeve"* or *"Pull up your pants."*

- Compliment the person with dementia about how he/she looks and the amount of effort demonstrated.

- Be flexible if the person with dementia wants to wear the same clothes two days in a row.

- Select clothing that is soft and comfortable on the person with dementia's skin.

- When possible, allow the person with dementia to select their favorite clothing or colors.

- Remove off-season clothing. For instance, remove shorts from the closet during the winter so that family member will not mistakenly put them on.

- Buy duplicates of the same outfit if the person with dementia insists on wearing the same clothes every day.

- Establish a social goal for dressing. For instance, tell the person with dementia a friend is coming to visit. Encouraged him/her to dress in an attractive manner.

Strategies to Manage Resistance to Eating

Changes to the Home Environment

- Arrange utensils, dishware and food in a consistent manner.

- Use a white plate to eliminate distractions from patterns on dishware.

- Keep the table setting simple by using one utensil. It may be easiest to have this utensil be a spoon, so that the person with dementia can scoop food up.

- Use a non-stick surface under a dish that has a color that contrasts with the dish.
  - For example, use a blue placement underneath a white dish.

- Use a travel mug with a non-spill top or a cup with a top and straw if spilling is a problem.

- Consider the use of cinnamon or orange potpourri to make foods smell appetizing.

- Use a shut-off switch on electrical or gas lines.

- Use assistive devices such as built up utensils or scoop dishes.

- Using a bowl, a scoop dish, or a plate with a plate guard will make it easier for the person with dementia to push their food onto their eating utensil.

- Using built-up utensils will make the utensils easier to grasp and hold on to.

- Use a large, stable eating surface in an area where the family normally eats.

- Adjust the height of tables or chairs to position the person with dementia optimally.

Changes to Eating Routines

- Present food items one at a time.

- Arrange food item attractively on the plate and table.

- Offer chopped or soft food if chewing is a problem.

- Moisten foods with gravy or sauce. Avoid foods with tough skins or food that falls apart in the mouth (nuts, seeds) and dry, sticky foods (white bread, peanut butter). Remember that even if it seems unappealing to you, the person with dementia may enjoy a food more when it's easy to chew and swallow.

- Cut food into small pieces if overstuffing is a problem.

- If overeating is a problem, place smaller portions on the plate.

- Check with the person with dementia's doctor and dentist for possible medical reasons for the person with dementia's reluctance to eat.
  - Talking with the person with dementia's health care professionals might give you insight about eating behaviors. In particular, you may want to:
  - Have the person with dementia's dentist check dentures and see if they still fit properly. If they do not, this will affect the person with dementia's ability to chew foods.

- Contact the person with dementia's physician or pharmacist to find out if any medications might interfere with appetite.

- Talk with the doctor about other conditions that could make it uncomfortable or difficult to eat, such as sores on the mouth or difficulty swallowing.

- Talk with the physician or a nutritionist about the extent to which you need to be concerned about the amount of food or liquids the person with dementia is consuming. They can help determine how many calories a day the person with dementia should be consuming. If the person with dementia is not as active as they once were, he or she might not require as much food now.

- Ask about snacks that have an effect on appetite and plan the person with dementia's snacks accordingly (e.g., caffeine can suppress appetite). If the person with dementia does not eat enough, try leaving nutritious snacks near the places where the person with dementia is most likely to sit during the day.

- Avoid arguing or trying to convince the person with dementia to eat if he or she refuses to eat. Arguing with or trying to convince people to eat can often lead to battles that are frustrating for both of you. The following suggestions might help:
  - Sit down to eat at the same time as the person with dementia.
  - Prompt occasionally if the person with dementia stops eating.
  - Be clear but specific in your prompts. For example, instead of asking him or her to eat, or explaining why they need to, simply say something like, *"Mom, please take a bite of potato."*
  - Be flexible. This will help keep both you and our family from becoming frustrated. For instance, if the person with dementia has difficulty eating one type of food, then try giving another type of food.

- Place a shirt, smock or apron on the person with dementia to catch food or drink spills.

- If a wheelchair is used, transfer to a "regular" chair when possible. If a wheelchair must be used at the table and the person with dementia can sit up easily, remove the wheelchair's arms.

- Position the person with dementia to provide a distance of 10 to 12 inches from plate to mouth.

- Use finger foods and encourage finger feeding if the person with dementia finds it difficult to use utensils.

- Finger foods can be nutritious and an easy alternative to having the person with dementia struggle with utensils. They can boost confidence in eating and maintain independent eating.

- Avoid eating while watching television. This may distract the person with dementia from eating.

- If you need to feed the person with dementia, use these feeding techniques:
  - Allow him/her sufficient time to swallow before another bite is introduced.
  - Do not overload the person with dementia's mouth.
  - Encourage the person with dementia to hold food/utensil and guide his/her hand to mouth.
  - Do not mix food into "hash."

- Use a light downward pressure on the chin to help get the person with dementia to open his/her mouth.
  - Gently remind the person with dementia to chew, eat slowly, and to swallow.
  - Stay at the table and eat with the person with dementia.

- If family members or friends who are not usually present are asked to share in a meal, try to appoint one familiar member to attend primarily to the social interaction needs of the person with dementia.

- If possible, keep the social group small (4 total, including you and the person with dementia).

- Use touch to help calm or stimulate the person with dementia as appropriate.

Strategies to Manage Resistance to Grooming (Personal Hygiene)

Changes to the Home Environment

- Place items for one specific grooming task in a marked container. Containers may be clear plastic or opaque and can be marked (from simplest to most complex):
  - a picture of the person with dementia performing the task for which the objects are needed
  - a drawing or picture of another person performing the task; a drawing of the objects; or a label indicating the task and/or objects (For example, all shaving items may be marked "Shaving Items" and include a picture of a person shaving. For individuals with reading comprehension problems, an actual photograph of the person with dementia shaving is preferred.)

- Remove objects that are not used by the person with dementia on a daily basis. Also remove from view all objects that belong to (an)other family member(s).

- Use only products and product packaging that are familiar to the person with dementia. For instance, pump-type containers of soap and toothpaste may be too new and too confusing.

- Purchase several identical personal care items at one time in order to have familiar replacements on hand. For instance, buy several toothbrushes or combs, all the same style and color, and use these to replace worn or lost items.

- Provide physical assistance with all electrical appliances used in the bathroom or arrange for the person with dementia to use those appliances in another room.

- When necessary, remove all electrical appliances from the bathroom.

- Adjust the hot water heater to no higher than 120 degrees in order to avoid burns.

- Use built-up grooming devices.

- Use bright hot colors (red, yellows and oranges) and/or large sizes or print to highlight instructions or items that are to be noticed.

Changes to Grooming Routines

- Do not ask the person with dementia if he/she wants to go brush teeth, shave, etc. Instead, tell them, *"Please, brush your teeth now."*

- Hand grooming items to the person with dementia as they are needed. Name each item as it is presented.

- Schedule the person with dementia's grooming for periods of the day when others in the household are not waiting for the bathroom. This will allow the person with dementia to take the necessary amount of time for grooming.

- Establish a social goal for good grooming, such as saying, *"You look so clean and nice. Let's go for a walk and show you off."*

Incontinence

What Is Incontinence?

Incontinence refers to loss of bladder and/or bowel control and/or bedwetting. One type of incontinence can occur without the other. Incontinence is common in the latter stages of the disease.

Why Might Incontinence Occur?

If incontinence is a new behavior, then the first step is to identify possible reasons for the loss of control. The incontinence may be due to a reversible medical condition. Even so, it may be possible to manage it by changing the person with dementia's routine, clothing, or environment.

Common Triggers

- Medical condition such as a urinary tract infection, constipation, or a prostate problem
- Difficulty getting to the bathroom in time due to impaired mobility
- Side effect of a medication
- Inability to find the bathroom
- Difficulty undressing when using the bathroom
- Not recognizing the urge to urinate
- Difficulty seeing or recognizing the toilet/commode
- Inability to express the need to use the bathroom

Strategies

Changes to the Home Environment

- Use a simple and straightforward picture or photograph of the toilet and place it in an area that the person with dementia will easily see when trying to locate the bathroom.

- Close all doors except the bathroom door.

- Paint the bathroom door a bright, eye-catching color.

- Use large arrows pointing the way to the bathroom from the living room or bedroom.

- Hang a drawing over the toilet of a man or woman using the toilet.

- Use a colored, padded toilet seat.

- Use a nightlight at night, or keep the bathroom light on at all times.

- Remove or cover containers in the bathroom such as the sink, wastebasket, or laundry hamper if the person with dementia uses these as a toilet.

- Use assistive devices to make the toileting process safer and easier:
  - Use grab bars for toilet transfers.
  - Use a raised toilet seat.
  - Use a commode in the bedroom for nighttime use.

Changes to Daily Routines

- Avoid blaming or scolding the person with dementia if he/she has an accident.
  - Remember that accidents are embarrassing.
  - Try to be matter-of-fact and understanding about accidents. When the person with dementia is successful, use praise and encouragement.

- Watch for visible cues that the person with dementia may need to use the bathroom.
  - Encourage the person with dementia to tell you when he or she needs to use the bathroom.
  - If he or she is unable to, look for signs such as unusual sounds or faces, restlessness, unzipping clothing, or pacing.

- Identify when accidents occur and plan ahead.

- Record the day and time of incontinence to establish a bathroom schedule.

- Establish a routine for toileting every two hours.

- If a toileting routine has been established, avoid unnecessary changes in that routine.

- Give instructions in the form of a statement, instead of a question. For example, *"Let's use the bathroom now"* rather than *"Do you have to use the toilet?"*

- Use body language, such as taking the person with dementia's elbow and walking toward and/or pointing toward the bathroom.

SECTION
7

- Consult with the person with dementia's doctor in case the incontinence is due to a medical condition.

- Reduce intake of alcohol and caffeine. These are potential bladder irritants and may make the person with dementia need to urinate more urgently or more often.

- Avoid liquids a few hours before bedtime.

- Physically help the person with dementia remove clothing and sit on the toilet.

- Keep the person with dementia's clothing simple and practical. Consider:
  - pants or skirts with elastic waistbands or Velcro openings
  - two-piece outfits so that only the soiled half needs to be changed

- Consider using such products as pads or protective bedding, adult diapers or panty liners for female patients.

- Stimulate urination by giving the person with dementia a drink of water or running water in the sink.

- Encourage the person with dementia (unless the doctor says otherwise) to drink six cups of fluids daily.

- For variety, try decaffeinated teas, decaffeinated coffee, Jell-O, Popsicles or fruit juice.

- If a fiber supplement is recommended, it should be given at the same time everyday to establish a routine.

- Remember that the incontinence is either due to a medical condition or the disease, and is not something the person with dementia can control.

Behaviors That Are Harmful to Self

What Are Behaviors That Are Harmful to Self?

Self-destructive behaviors may be intentional or unintentional. Intentionally or deliberately inflicted behaviors such as self-cutting can result in pain or injury. Other behaviors are more indirectly or unintentionally self-destructive. Examples of this include not taking medications, driving, leaving the stove burner on, or not eating properly. Individuals may be unaware that these behaviors are dangerous to themselves and can be very upsetting.

Why Might Behaviors That Are Harmful to Self Occur?

Most people with dementia do not recognize their own impairments. They also do not recognize the risk or potential harm of an action. In addition, some types of dementia produce "La belle indifference," an inability to experience worry, concern or anxiety.

Common Triggers

- Depression
- Inability to use equipment appropriately
- Inability to recognize or accurately perceive objects
- Not realizing that the behavior is dangerous to themselves

Strategies

- Lock up or dispose of dangerous objects. These include such items as matches, knives, lighters, power tools, irons and guns.

- Dispose of all old medications. This is so that the person with dementia does not mistakenly take them.

- Check batteries on smoke detectors and make sure the alarm is loud enough to easily be heard. Keep a fire extinguisher in the kitchen.

- Lower the temperature on your hot water heater. This way the person with dementia cannot accidentally scald themselves.

- Limit access to potentially dangerous areas such as the basement or shed by locking doors if the person tends to wander.

- Lock up or dispose of toxic materials. Toxic materials include cleaning fluids, insecticides and medicines. This is so that they are not accidentally ingested by the person with dementia. Medications can be kept in a locked box, cabinet or drawer.

- Learn to disable the car if the person with dementia insists on driving.

- Remove poisonous plants (like oleander) so they are not mistakenly eaten.

- Remove knobs from the stove so that the person with memory loss cannot switch it on. If you have an electric stove, you can install a switch on the back of the stove so that when the switch is off, the burners will not work.

- Secure exits, including doors and windows, so that the person with dementia does not hurt him/herself.

- Install child safety latches on the inside of cabinets where cleaning products are kept.

- Remove locks from doors where the person with dementia could accidentally lock themselves inside a room.

- Post important numbers by the telephone: police, fire, family and friends.
  - If you own a phone on which numbers may be programmed, program the emergency numbers. This will save time in case of an emergency.

- Distract or re-direct the person with dementia.

- This could involve playing a simple game, listening to soothing music, or looking at family photograph albums.

- Provide the person with dementia with more supervision. This might mean enrolling the person with dementia in an adult day service a few days a week, or having someone stay with him/her in the home for a portion of the day.

- Talk with the person with dementia's doctor. Depression should be considered, especially if the person you are caring for talks about suicide and attempts to hurt him/herself. Consider a discussion with the doctor about antidepressant medication. Such drugs are being used for depression in dementia with good results.

Destroying Property

What Is Destroying Property?

People with dementia sometimes damage or destroy things as a result of their inability to move their body appropriately or use items (e.g., utensils) correctly. The inability to initiate and execute movements is called apraxia, and it is extremely common in dementia. Identifying possible triggers for agitation is the key to preventing catastrophic reactions.

Why Might Property Destruction Occur?

Identify possible triggers for the agitation. This is the key to preventing catastrophic reactions.

Common Triggers

- No longer understands how to use the item
- Agitation that has led to anger and frustration
- Catastrophic reaction

Strategies

- Keep especially fragile items out of sight.

- Tools like hammers or knives should also be safeguarded. This will help prevent the person with dementia from using them and possibly causing damage.

- Managing the agitation that may lead to the destruction of property:
  - Distract the person with dementia and re-direct him or her to another activity.
  - Move the person with dementia into a more soothing environment.
  - Use a calm and reassuring voice.

- Set up a room in which the person with dementia can safely "tinker."
  - This room might have drawers the person with dementia can open and close, can take things out of, and can put things into.

Sexually Inappropriate Behavior

What Is Sexually Inappropriate Behavior?

Inappropriate sexual behavior may take various forms:

- Masturbating in the bedroom with the door open

- Removing clothes and exposing self in public places or to neighbors

- Groping one's spouse in public

- Behaving sexually toward strangers in public places (e.g., waitresses in restaurants)

Why Might Sexually Inappropriate Behavior Occur?

Sexual feelings normally continue into late life and into dementia. In some types of dementia, sexual feelings or their expression may be exaggerated. The term for this is hypersexuality. A common problem that complicates hypersexuality in dementia is disinhibition, the loss of normal inhibitions or judgment. These behaviors can be very distressing to the person you care for. Social graces may deteriorate, and the person may make inappropriate comments in public. People often lack insight into the consequences of their behavior as well. The behaviors have a physical cause, and are not usually something that the person can control or contain.

Common Triggers

- Misunderstanding of the need to be undressed for bathing
- Misinterpretation of a hug as sexual contact
- Uncomfortable — too warm, clothing too tight
- Genital irritation
- Need to urinate
- Need for attention, affection, intimacy
- Self-stimulating, reacting to what feels good
- Groin rash or irritation
- Stool impaction
- Alcohol abuse/withdrawal

Strategies to Prevent Sexually Inappropriate Behavior

- Put the person's clothes (especially pants) on backwards, or put the belt buckle in the back. This will help prevent the person you care for from disrobing in public.

- Monitor and turn off TV programs with sexual content (e.g., afternoon soap operas).

- Inform the doctor about the person's sexual behavior (if you think it isn't normal), and find out if there is any medical management that may be tried.

- Avoid the social outings where the inappropriate behavior occurs.

- If the person with dementia is your spouse, and if you do not wish to have sex with him or her, change bedroom or change time of retiring (let him or her go to sleep first) or time of rising in the morning (before the person you care for gets up).

- Do not give mixed sexual messages, even in jest.

- Avoid nonverbal sexual messages.

- Distract the person with dementia while performing personal care such as bathing by talking about something else.

- Check room temperature to determine if too warm.

- Introduce comfortable clothing.

Strategies to Use If Sexually Inappropriate Behavior Occurs

- Use an explanation card to give to strangers who may be approached by the person you care for, in order to explain about his/her inappropriate behavior.

- Respond calmly and firmly. Do not overreact or confront. If the person you care for is undressed in a public place or the front yard, offer him/her a robe to put on, or walk with him/her to a more secluded area to handle the situation.

- Use distraction and redirection.

- Introduce exercise.

- Introduce soft music to create a calm environment.

Socially Inappropriate Behavior

What Is Socially Inappropriate Behavior?

Changes in the social behavior of individuals with dementia are very common. People with dementia do not follow social rules about what or where to say or do something. For example, a person with dementia might comment tactlessly about someone else's appearance. These behaviors can be very upsetting for caregivers.

Why Might Socially Inappropriate Behavior Occur?

Disinhibition, the loss of normal judgment or tact, is the cause of the inappropriate behaviors. Disinhibited behaviors are those words or actions which seem tactless, rude or offensive.

Common Triggers

- Disorientation
- Confusion (e.g., mistaking a daughter for a wife)
- Asking a person to do a task that is too complicated

Strategies to Prevent Socially Inappropriate Behavior

- Limit contact with strangers; there are still ways to engage in your regular activities while reducing the chances something embarrassing will occur. For example, go to restaurants in their non-peak hours and find a quiet booth to sit in. If the person with dementia needs to go with you to the grocery store, try to find a time when it will not be too crowded.

- Prepare a simple explanation or carry pre-written explanation cards to give to strangers if the person with dementia does something that is socially inappropriate.

- Do not argue with the person with dementia. Let the person you care for know that the behavior bothers you by using a soft voice and calming words. Reassure him or her if they appear lost, confused or frightened. Try to speak slowly and clearly so that the person you care for will understand you.

- Be prepared to communicate your requests and intentions repeatedly. The person with dementia may not understand what you are requesting immediately. Also, the person you care for might also forget that you have asked him or her not to do or say something.

- Try not to take the words or actions of the person you care for personally. Remember that it is the disease that is causing the inappropriate behavior.

- Engage the person you care for in an activity. For instance, if you see the person you care for talking to someone in the grocery store, calmly go over to him or her and remind them that they need to stay with you while you are shopping. Then ask him or her to assist you in some way, such as by pushing the shopping cart or holding a box of cereal.

SECTION
7

Aggressive or Combative Behaviors (Verbally or Physically Threatening Behavior)

What Are Combative Behaviors?

Combative behaviors can be either physical or verbal in nature. Aggression usually builds up in stages, with anxiety being exhibited first, progressing toward verbal behaviors. Verbally combative behaviors refer to negative verbal outbursts. If these behaviors are not effectively dealt with, they can advance to physically combative behavior. Physically combative behaviors refer to physical actions such as hitting, pushing, pinching or pulling hair.

Why Might Combative Behaviors Occur?

Agitation and combative behaviors can be triggered or provoked by similar factors in the environment. People with dementia often cannot understand what is happening around them and may find the actions or words of those around them bothersome. Their disinhibition may prevent their recognizing the consequences of their behavior.

Common Triggers

- Pain or discomfort
- Lack of rest or sleep
- Eyesight or hearing problems
- Side effects of medicines such as nervousness or paranoia
- Too much going on in the environment
- Unfamiliar surroundings
- Change in routine
- Picking up on your stress and frustration
- Fear
- Loss of control due to changes in the brain
- Being told to do something they no longer know how to do
- Communication deficits
- Medical problems
- Physical restraints

Strategies to Minimize Combative Behaviors

Changes to the Home Environment

- Avoid places with loud noise or too much activity. Too many people and physical clutter should also be avoided.

- Keep familiar objects: pictures, stuffed animals, favorite clothes or a soft cloth may have a calming effect on the person with dementia.

- Also, favorite pets may be calming.

- Avoid making changes in your home when you can. For example, try to leave a favorite chair or one used by the person you care for in the same place. If you do make changes, make them gradually.

Steps to Prevent Frustration

- Be reasonable about your expectations of what the person you care for can do.

- He or she will not be able to do all the things they could before.

- Plan stressful activities for when the person with dementia is most rested.

- You may want to give a bath shortly after the person you care for gets up and has breakfast.

- Make sure the person you care for gets plenty of rest.

- See that the person you care for gets exercise. For example, take a daily walk with him or her.

- If the person you care for has failed to complete or carry out a task, do not press him to continue trying.

- Distract the person you care for and try again later.

Establish a Routine

- Do the same things at the same time each day.

- Limit the number of choices to avoid confusion. For example, let the person with dementia choose between two pairs of pants instead of ten.

- Break tasks into parts and give step-by-step instructions.

- Allow the person with dementia to finish a step before you give another.

- Validate the person with dementia. Offer support and acceptance for what the person with dementia believes, even if it is different or doesn't go along with your reality.

- Do not rationalize with the person with dementia. People with dementia really believe what they say; trying to convince them they are wrong will only make them more upset. It may be better to agree or change the subject.

- Try to be flexible if you know a certain situation is likely to upset the person with dementia. For example, the person with dementia may become agitated when preparing for bed. Try to make this time as short and pleasant as possible.

- Never approach the person with dementia quickly.

- Don't startle the person with dementia; always approach from the front.

- Pay attention to your body language. The person with dementia may pick up on anger and frustration you are feeling. Try to avoid putting your hands on your hips, frowning, or pointing a finger at the person with dementia.

- Do not ask too many questions or make too many statements at once.

- Try to get the person with dementia to tell you if he or she is upset. This way you will have a better idea of what you should do.

Keep Frustration from Getting Out of Hand

- Watch for signs of frustration, such as fidgeting, restlessness and loud talking.

- Once you have identified a sign, you can try to prevent the situation from getting worse.

- Respond to anger and outbursts in a calm and direct manner. You may be able to prevent an angry episode from getting worse.

- State clearly and in an even tone, *"You are safe here; nobody is going to hurt you."* Repeat frequently and calmly until the behavior stops.

- If the person with dementia becomes upset while trying to finish a task, try another task. Return to the first task when the person with dementia is no longer upset.

- If the person with dementia becomes upset while putting on socks, take a break and brush their hair. Once the person with dementia has calmed down, try putting the socks on again.

- Determine whether anger or agitation is due to physical (i.e., medical) or environmental causes.

- If possible, take the person with dementia away from an upsetting situation. Take him or her to a quiet room or go for a walk.

- Avoid confrontation.

- Try to distract the person with dementia or offer an alternative activity, such as suggesting you look at a photo album or have a cup of tea together.

- Respect the person with dementia's personal space.

- The person with dementia might feel more comfortable if you stay at arms length from them. If you come too close, the person may feel threatened, become angry, or strike out.

When the Angry Outburst Is Over

- Do not blame the person with dementia after an episode of acting out. The person with dementia most likely will not remember the behavior.

- Try not to take the person with dementia's outburst personally. He or she was probably frustrated or confused.

- Pay special attention to the situation and what may have caused the problem. You may be able to see a pattern or determine a cause. Keep a record of outbursts and look for a pattern. Note what happened, who was present at the time, and what happened just before the combative episode. This will help you avoid such problems in the future.

- Give the person with dementia some time to him/herself. This will give him/her some time to cool down before you approach them again.

Worrying, Fearfulness, Anxiety and Depression

What Are Worrying, Fearfulness, Anxiety and Depression?

These are common feelings that may emerge as the dementia progresses. While people with dementia may not express these feelings directly, they may appear very sad or lethargic. They may wring their hands nervously or follow family caregivers around the house.

Why Might These Feelings Occur?

These feelings may be an expression of underlying fear and anxiety as to what is happening to them or confusion as to where they are.

Common Triggers

- Response to loss of abilities which the person with dementia may sense, especially early in the disease

- Sense of disorientation or confusion; this in turn may produce anxiety and fear

- Physical changes in the brain

- Side effect of a medication

- Physical illness

- Social isolation

- Fatigue

- Inability to screen out unwanted stimulation such as loud noises and crowds

Strategies to Help Manage Fears and Suffering

- Try to maintain a daily routine.

- Allow the person with dementia to express his or her feelings.

- If the person with dementia can express feelings verbally, give him or her chances to talk about being worried or anxious. Listen to him or her and provide comfort.

- If the person you care for has difficulty expressing emotions verbally, try asking him or her to point to a picture that shows how he or she is feeling.

- If that does not work, begin to guess. Say, "Are you worried? Nod your head if you feel worried."

- Offer a snack or a drink that is a "comfort food" for the person you care for.

- Do not mention leaving before you need to.

- Play soothing music.

- Try a hug, gentle back or arm rub, holding hands, or some other form of touching that might bring comfort.

- Speak in a calm and reassuring tone of voice. You might say, "You look worried today. Remember that I am here to help."

- Be positive, as frequent praise will help both you and the person you care for feel better.

- Determine whether large group situations cause the person you care for to feel worse, or whether he or she benefits from the stimulation of a busy, active gathering.

- It is important to know what the person has enjoyed in the past, as it is likely that similar activities will still appeal now.

- Provide activities for the person you care for to participate in.

- Empty time may lead to mood or behavior problems. Although the person you care for may find some activities frustrating, it is important to keep him/her engaged in activities that he or she can do. The person you care for may be able to do certain things with some help. Some chores may be enjoyable. Staying busy and having fun will help to support the person with dementia's mood. Create activities based on past hobbies and interests, and think of the strengths and weaknesses of the person you care for. Pick activities that use his or her strengths. Avoid those that require capabilities he or she no longer has.

- Scheduling some pleasant events into each day's activities may help to improve the person with dementia's mood. These may be simple activities like taking a walk, gardening, listening to music, or talking to friends or relatives on the phone. You can make games like dominoes or cards easier, using big dominoes or just simplifying the game.

- Talk to the doctor of the person you care for. Treatment of depression and by many antidepressants, especially the SSRI drugs (specific serotonin re-uptake inhibitors), is often very successful in people with dementia. Depression is often accompanied by anxiety, and often both can be treated with the same medication. There are also medications that can make the situation worse, so it is always best to report what you see to the doctor.

- Be aware of when the person with dementia is the least tired and do important tasks at that time.

- Have the person with dementia talk to a professional counselor. Psychotherapy, either individual or group therapy, may be available for people in early-stage dementia. Medicare now reimburses for psychotherapy for people with dementia.

Distressing Beliefs: Seeing, Hearing or Sensing Things

What Are Distressing Beliefs?

People with memory loss sometimes experience hallucinations or delusions. Hallucinations are things the person senses that are not there. He or she may see, hear, smell, taste or feel these things. Delusions are beliefs about something that are false. Often the person cannot be persuaded that the idea is wrong. Although hallucinations and delusions are imaginary, they seem very real and can cause extreme anxiety, even panic.

Why Might Distressing Beliefs Occur?

Impairments in visual perception, caused by the dementia, may cause someone to believe he/she has seen someone who was not in fact there. Impaired comprehension also produces delusions or hallucinations.

Common Triggers

- Dark or unwelcoming environment; uneven lighting that causes shadows
- Physical conditions such as infections, fever, pain, constipation or dehydration
- Forgetting where they put something (such as a wallet)
- Disruption of familiar routines
- Unfamiliar people
- Side effects of medication
- Poor vision or hearing
- Too much noise or activity

SECTION

7

Strategies

- Ignore hallucinations or delusions that are not bothering the person with dementia. For example, the person you care for may believe they are talking to a relative who has died, or they hear pleasant music. This may bring comfort to the person you care for.

- Avoid arguing with the person you care for about what he or she sees or hears.

- It is better to acknowledge that the person you care for may be frightened by the delusions and hallucinations.

- Respond to the feeling he or she is expressing and provide reassurance and comfort.

- Turn off the television set, especially when violent or disturbing programs are on.

- The person you care for may not be able to distinguish what he or she sees on television from reality.

- Try to distract the person you care for to another topic or activity.

- Sometimes moving to another room or going outside for a walk may help.

- Make sure the person you care for is safe and does not have access to anything that could cause harm to him/herself or anyone else.

- nvestigate suspicions to make sure they are not founded on fact.

- Consult the physician of the person you care for with regard to:
  - review of medications for possible causes
  - underlying medical causes
  - underlying vision or hearing problems
  - potential medications to treat delusions if the person you care becomes violent or threatening

Changes in the Home Environment

- Maintain a consistent daily routine and try to maintain consistent caregivers (such as home health aides).

- Ensure adequate lighting in the areas used by the person you care for; keep a night-light on at night.

- Use physical touch to reassure the person you care for.

- Provide reassurance that the person you care for is safe.

- Make sure the eyeglasses of the person you care for are clean and/or the hearing aid is working properly.

- Regulate the amount and type of social interactions that the person you care for has (number of people coming into the home).

Sleep Disturbances

What Are Sleep Disturbances?

- People with memory loss often experience difficulty sleeping.

- Sleep disturbances may include an inability to fall asleep, an inability to stay asleep, waking up throughout the night and/or wandering, becoming agitated at night and/or having distressful thoughts that awaken the person.

Why Might Sleep Disturbances Occur?

- Physiological or medical causes may include pain, underlying illness (diabetes, congestive heart failure) or infection (urinary tract infection), depression or side effects of medication.

- Environmental causes may include room temperature (too hot or too cold), lighting (too much or too little), noise (television, radio, noise from others coming and going), or a change in the environment (as from home to hospital).

- Other causes may include too much sleeping/napping during the day, being agitated or upset about something that happened in the day, not enough physical activity, too much caffeine or alcohol, hunger, and disturbing thoughts, beliefs or dreams.

Common Triggers

- Unwelcoming or uncomfortable environment
- Uneven lighting that causes shadows
- Physical conditions such as infections, fever, pain or hunger
- Too much fluids, especially caffeine or alcohol
- Inadequate physical exercise throughout the day
- Side effects of medication
- Poor vision or hearing
- Too much noise or activity in the environment

Strategies

- Consult with a doctor to determine if medications, an underlying medical problem, pain, restless legs or sleep apnea (difficulty breathing) are contributing to the sleep disturbances.

- Consult with doctor to determine if a medication that causes sleeplessness can be taken in the morning.

- Establish a predictable daily routine that includes opportunities for physical activity.

- Stop intake of caffeinated beverages (coffee, tea and soft drinks) or chocolate by 5:00 p.m. or earlier in the day.

- Determine if the environment is conducive to sleeping (e.g., not too dark or too light, quiet).

- Establish a bedtime routine that may include a quiet activity such as listening to soothing music.

- Safeproof the house if night wandering occurs (e.g., using locks, alarms or bells on doors to outside so that you are alerted; removing dangerous items or blocking off kitchen/stove; removing gates from stairs to keep person from climbing over or falling over).

- Avoid arguing with the person with dementia or talking about what will happen the next day.

- Try to prevent napping throughout the day. However, if necessary, have person only take a short rest or nap early in the day.

- Turn off the television set, especially when violent or disturbing programs are on.

Changes in the Home Environment

- Maintain a consistent daily routine and try to maintain consistent caregivers (such as home health aides).

- Ensure adequate lighting in the areas the person with dementia uses; keep a night-light on at night.

- Use physical touch to reassure the person with dementia.

- Provide reassurance that the person with dementia is safe.

- Make sure the person with dementia's eyeglasses are clean and/or the hearing aid is working properly and placed near the bedside.

Worksheets

Stress Diary

Try different stress reduction techniques to see which one works best for you. It is also important to keep practicing these techniques. The more you use a strategy that you like, the more effective it will be in helping to relieve your stress. Also, try to keep a record of the situations you find most stressful and how the different stress reduction techniques work for you in these situations. The "Stress Diary" can help you keep track. Before and after you use the technique, rate your tension level using this scale:

1 = Not at all tense
2 = Slightly tense
3 = Moderately tense
4 = Really tense
5 = Terribly tense

Date	Situation	Level of Tension	Comments
		Before: After:	
		Before: After:	
		Before: After:	
		Before: After:	
		Before: After:	

Behaviors That Are Challenging

Behavioral symptoms are a hallmark of any of the dementias. They can occur at any time and across the disease progression. Most people with dementia will experience one or more behaviors. Using structured routines and activities can help prevent behavioral symptoms yet some behaviors may still occur. Some behaviors may be more challenging for you to address than others. Use this worksheet to describe the behaviors you find challenging and track when they occur.

Look for patterns and underlying causes of the behavior that can be modified or changed. Do you see any patterns? Does the behavior occur at a particular time of day? When people are at home? At night? Refer to the strategies in this guide to identify ways to address the behavior. Share this worksheet with health professionals and other family members as they may have helpful suggestions as to how best to address the behaviors.

Date	Describe behavior	List times of day behavior occurs	What happens before the behavior occurs?	What happens after the behavior occurs?

General Considerations for Using Activities

You can post this tipsheet on your refrigerator or where you can easily refer to it on a regular basis. It is a handy tool to help you remember how to use activities every day.

Simplify the area

- Set up a comfortable place for the activity and remove unnecessary objects.
- Reduce distractions (TV or radio).
- Be sure there is adequate lighting for the activity.

Simplify the activity

- Set up the activity ahead of time.
- Use simple materials that are bright with contrasting colors.
- Label objects as necessary.
- Limit the number of steps in the activity.

Enhance participation

- Choose activities that are repetitive and/or familiar.
- Provide verbal or physical assistance to avoid frustration.
- Use encouragement and praise.
- Remember—there is no right or wrong way.

Communicate effectively

- Use a calm voice.
- Use simple 1- or 2-step instructions.
- Avoid negative statements—remain positive.

As Abilities Change – Modify the Activity

The abilities of the person with dementia may change, making it difficult for him/her to participate in activities that were previously enjoyed.

Keep simplifying the activity

- Reduce the number of materials used.
- Reduce the steps needed to complete an activity.
- Simplify instructions—use touch and demonstration.

Use passive activities

- Video
- Music
- Looking at photos

Change your expectations—Relax the rules—Focus on strengths

Notes:

How to Encourage Participation by Making an Activity Easier

As the abilities of a person with dementia change over time, you may need to simplify the activity to enable continued participation. Use this worksheet to list the particular activity and brainstorm ways to make it easier. For example, if the person with dementia enjoys making a salad but is no longer able to safely cut the ingredients, you could buy precut ingredients, or cut ingredients yourself and place in small containers and have the person assemble the salad. Or, let's say the person likes to make beaded necklaces but is now unable to place the beads on the string. You could have the person sort beads by colors instead. These are a few examples of ways to change an activity so that it fits better with what a person with dementia can do and participate in.

List Each Activity	List Ways to Simplify the Activity

Make Everyday Life Easier

Use this worksheet to identify the specific care challenges you have and identify strategies in this guide that may be helpful. By listing potential strategies on this worksheet, you can refer to it daily and also more easily share these tips with other family members.

List the Care Challenge	List Ways to Make It Better

Notes

What strategies are effective?

What strategies are not effective?

What strategies or activities would you like to consider now or in the future?

SECTION
8